Primal Safety Coloring Book

We hope you will use this coloring book to talk to your family about how you stay safe when you are at work. It is our belief that everyone should go home safely with no injuries at the end of each work day. You may also use this book to raise safety awareness on your jobsite. Bring your kid's colored pages in, laminate them, and put them up around the jobsite. Have a coloring contest with prizes. Use these pages to start safety discussions.

The Primal Safety Program is in the back of this book. If you would like to know more about how emotional intelligence can not only make your projects safer, but transform your people and your company, please visit our website at *www.brentdarnell.com*.

All illustrations are by Jean Archambault. He can be reached at *archambault.jean@ me.com*.

Layout by Tudor Maier

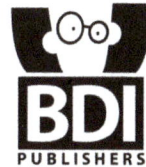

BDI
PUBLISHERS

Note: All profits from The Primal Safety Coloring Book go to help prevent suicide in the construction industry in the name of Bob A. Darnell, my father, who passed away in March of 2009.

According to the CDC, Construction has the second highest number of suicides than any other industry. It is estimated that suicides kill nine times more workers than the fatal four (falls, electrocution, struck by, caught in-between) accidents combined. As such, it is an industry imperative to shatter the mental health stigma and create caring cultures within our companies. The Construction Financial Management Association (CFMA) has established the Construction Industry Alliance for Suicide Prevention with the goal of providing and disseminating information and resources for suicide prevention and mental health promotion in construction. Through the information and resources CFMA has compiled, the Alliance looks to help those in the construction industry create awareness.

1

Libro para colorear sobre la seguridad primordial

Esperamos que usen este libro de colorear para hablar con su familia sobre cómo pueden mantenerse fuera de peligro cuando están trabajando. Creemos que al final de cada día laboral todos deben regresar a casa, sanos y salvos y sin ningunas heridas. Este libro lo pueden usar también para aumentar sus conocimientos sobre la seguridad en la obra de su proyecto. Traigan las páginas coloreadas por sus hijos, pónganlas con láminas y en la obra de su trabajo. Organicen un concurso de colorear con premios. Usen estas páginas para entablar unas conversaciones sobre la seguridad en el trabajo.

El Programa de Seguridad Primordial se encuentra en la parte posterior de este libro. Si desea saber más acerca de cómo la inteligencia emocional no sólo puede hacer que sus proyectos sean más seguros, sino que también puede transformar a su gente y a su empresa, visite nuestro sitio web en *www.brentdarnell.com*.

Todas las ilustraciones son de Jean Archambault. Puede ser contactado en *archambault.jean@me.com*. Diseño de interior y de cubierta: Tudor Maier

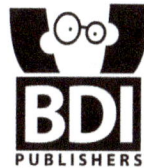

BDI
PUBLISHERS

Nota: Todos los beneficios de The Primal Safety Coloring Book se destinan a ayudar a prevenir el suicidio en la industria de la construcción a nombre de Bob A. Darnell, mi padre, que falleció en marzo de 2009.

De acuerdo a la CDC, la construcción presenta el segundo mayor numero de suicidios en comparación con otro tipo de industria. Se estima que los suicidios matan nueve veces más trabajadores que la combinación de los cuatros accidentes fatales (caídas, electrocución, golpes, quedar atrapados en el medio de materiales de construcción). Por lo tanto, en este tipo de industria es necesario romper con el estigma mental y crear una cultura de cuidado dentro de nuestras compañías. La Asociación de Gestión Financiera de la Construcción (o CFMA en sus siglas en ingles) ha establecido la Alianza de la industria de la Construcción para la prevención del suicidio, con el fin de proporcionar, difundir información y recursos para la prevención del suicidio y la promoción de la salud mental en la construcción. Por medio de la información y los recursos compilados por la CFMA, la Alianza busca tanto ayudar como crear conciencia en las personas que trabajan en el sector de la construcción.

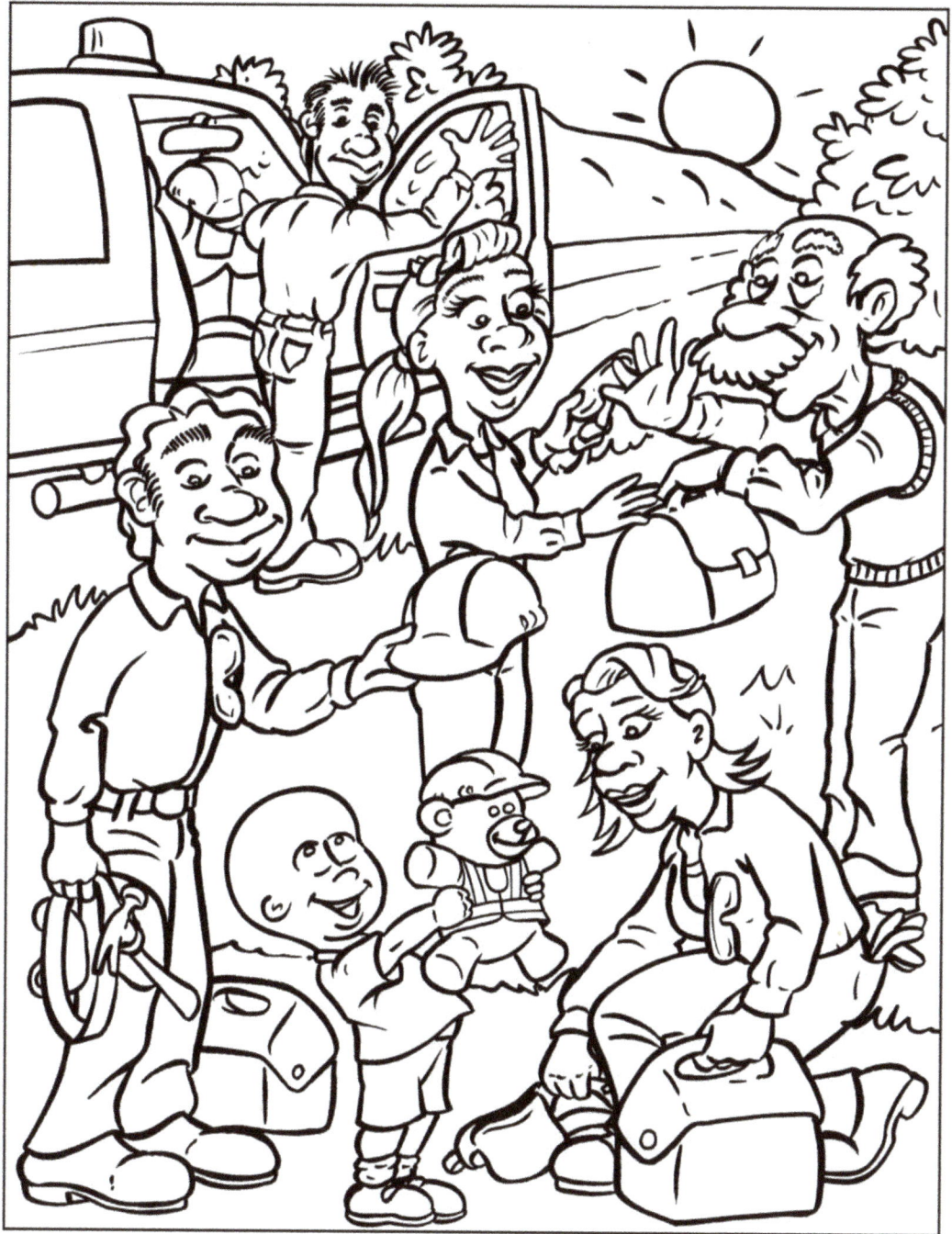

Everybody in my family builds things.
It's very exciting work, but it can be dangerous.

En mi familia todos construyen cosas.
Es un trabajo muy estimulante, pero puede ser peligroso.

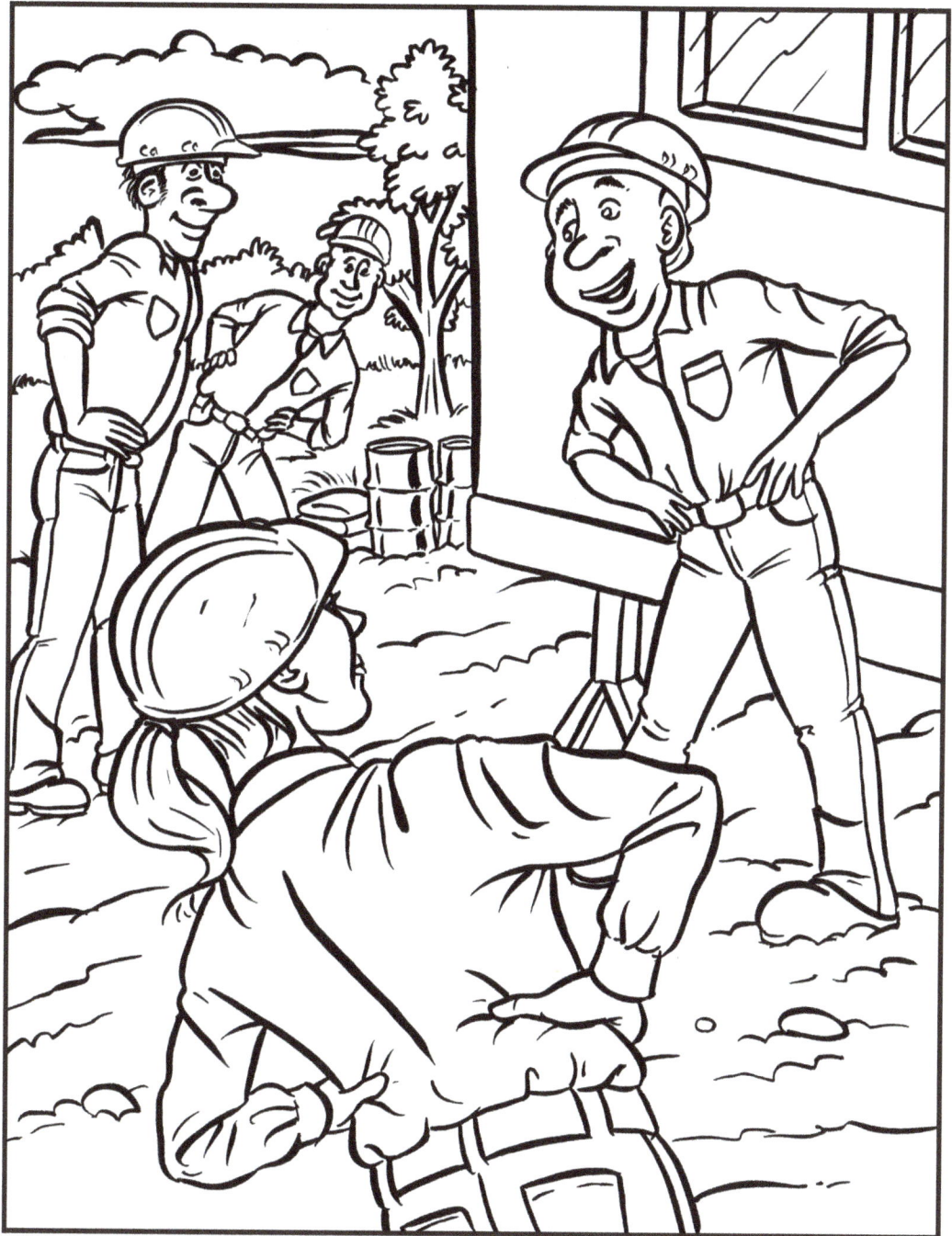

My dad helps to reduce injuries and increase safety
by leading everyone in morning stretches.

*Mi Papá ayuda a reducir las lesiones y a aumentar la seguridad
dirigiendo a todos en los estiramientos matutinos."*

4

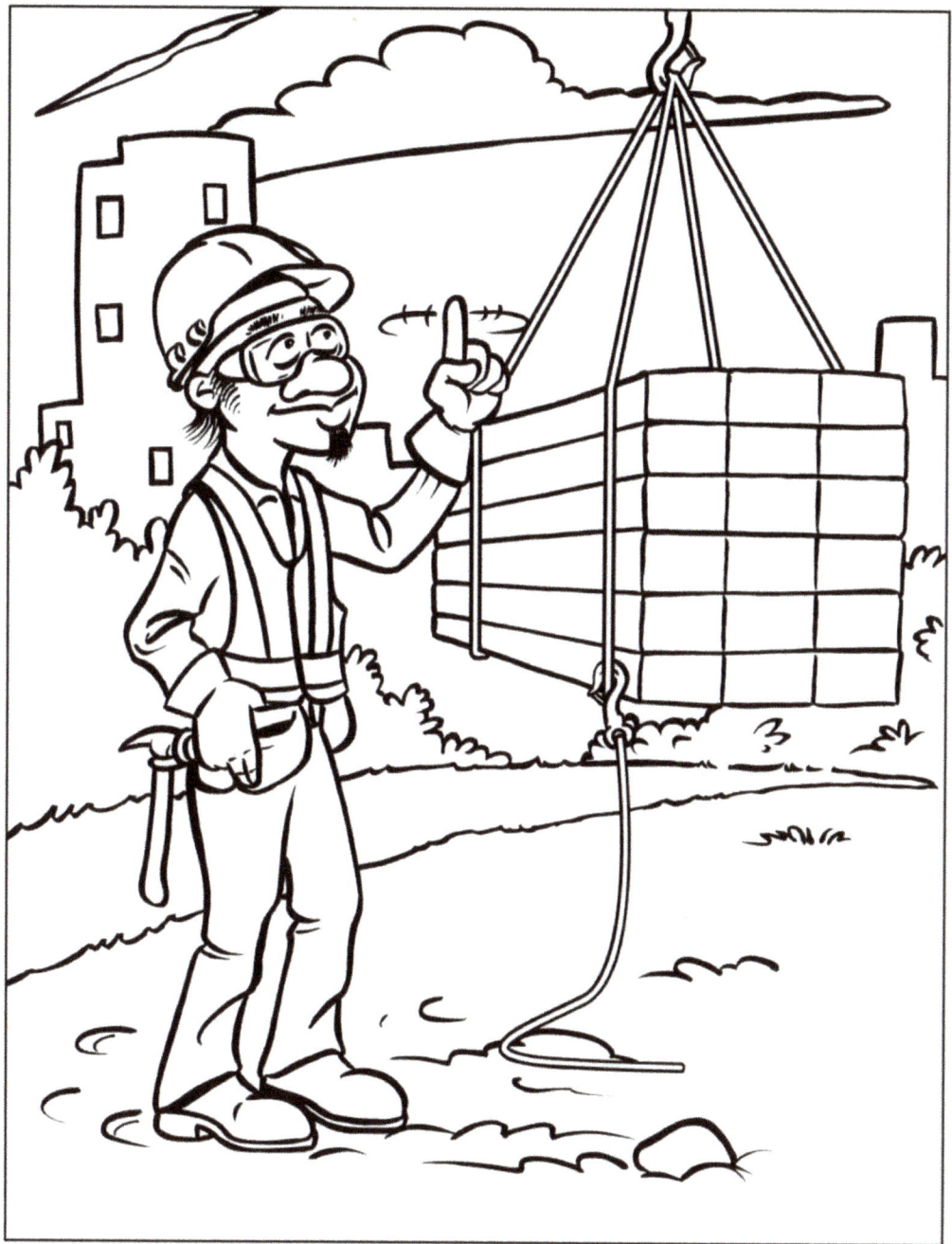

My brother always wears a bright vest so that people can see him, and he puts on the right shoes to protect his feet, and his hardhat to protect his head.

Mi hermano siempre lleva puesto un chaleco de un color vivo para que la gente lo vea, y también se pone los zapatos correctos para protegerse los pies y un casco para protegerse la cabeza.

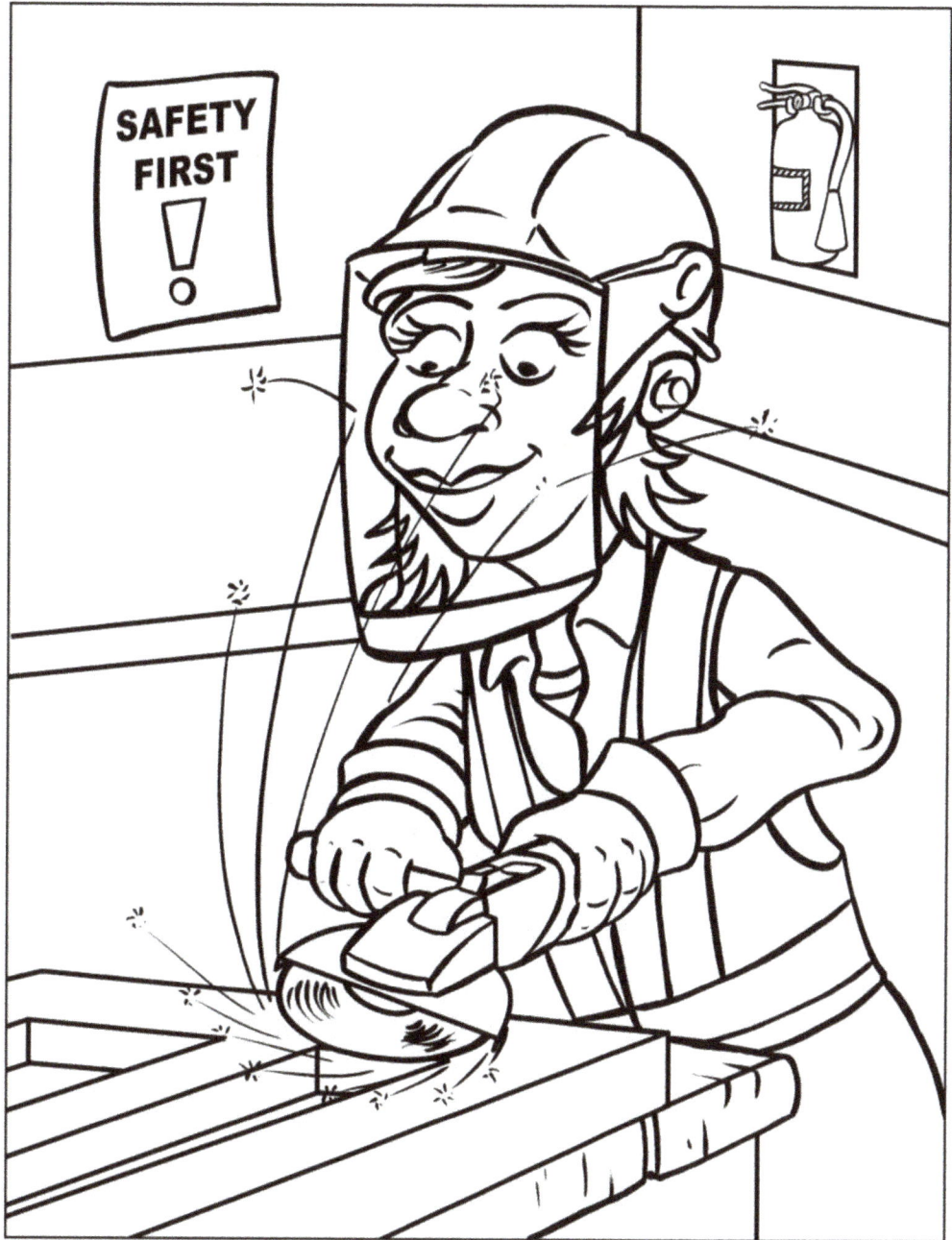

My mom always wears eye protection
so that her eyes won't get hurt.

*Mi mamá siempre lleva puesta alguna protección
para que no se le dañen los ojos.*

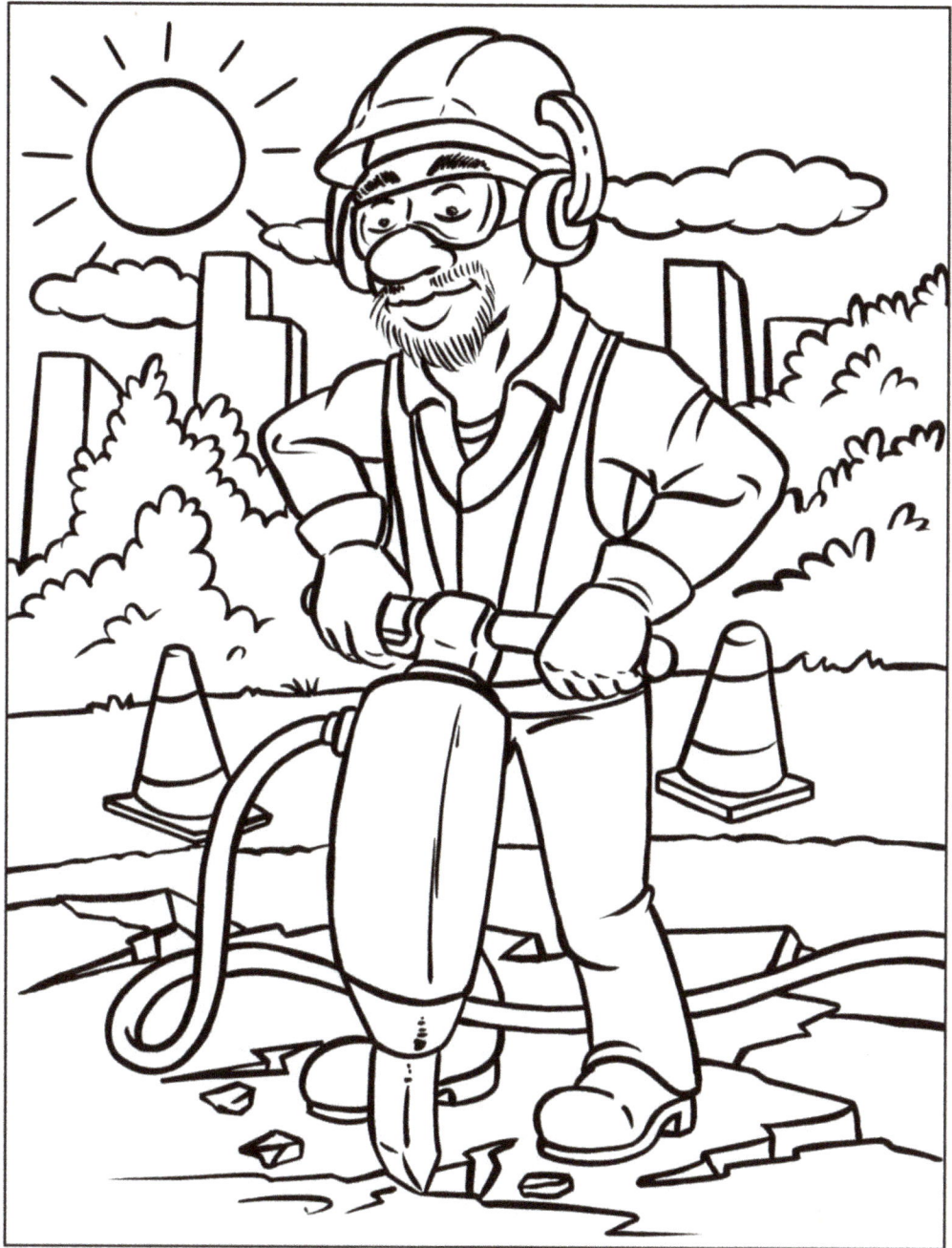

My uncle wears ear plugs when he's around loud noises
so that he protects his hearing.

*Cuando mi tío está en un lugar con ruidos fuertes siempre se pone tapones
en los oídos para protegerse la audición.*

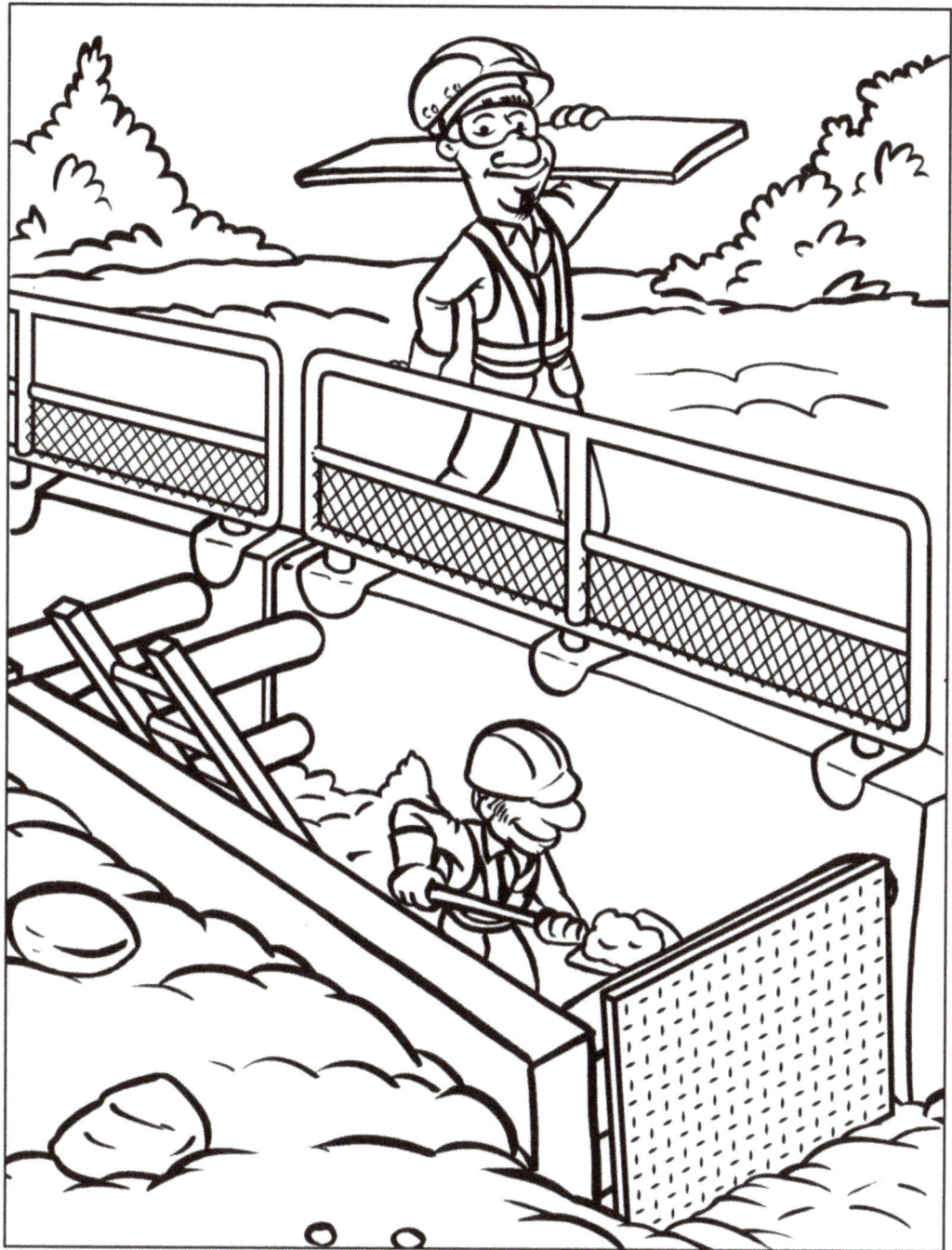

My brother is always careful when working
in or around a hole in the ground.

*Mi hermano siempre va con cuidado cuando está trabajando
cerca de o dentro de un agujero en el piso.*

8

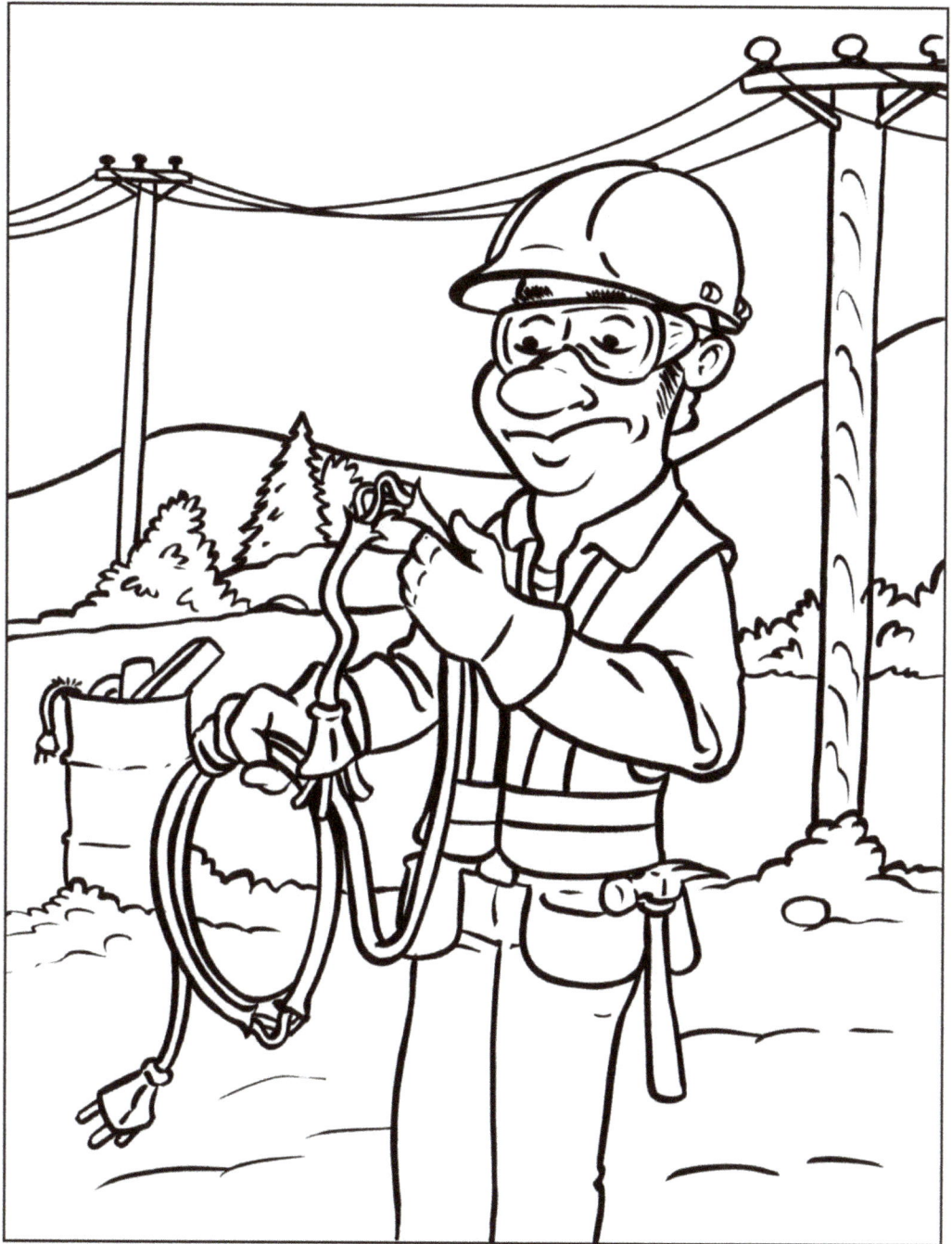

If my dad sees any electrical cords that are damaged,
he throws them away.

*Si ve mi papá algún que otro cordón eléctrico dañado,
se deshace de él.*

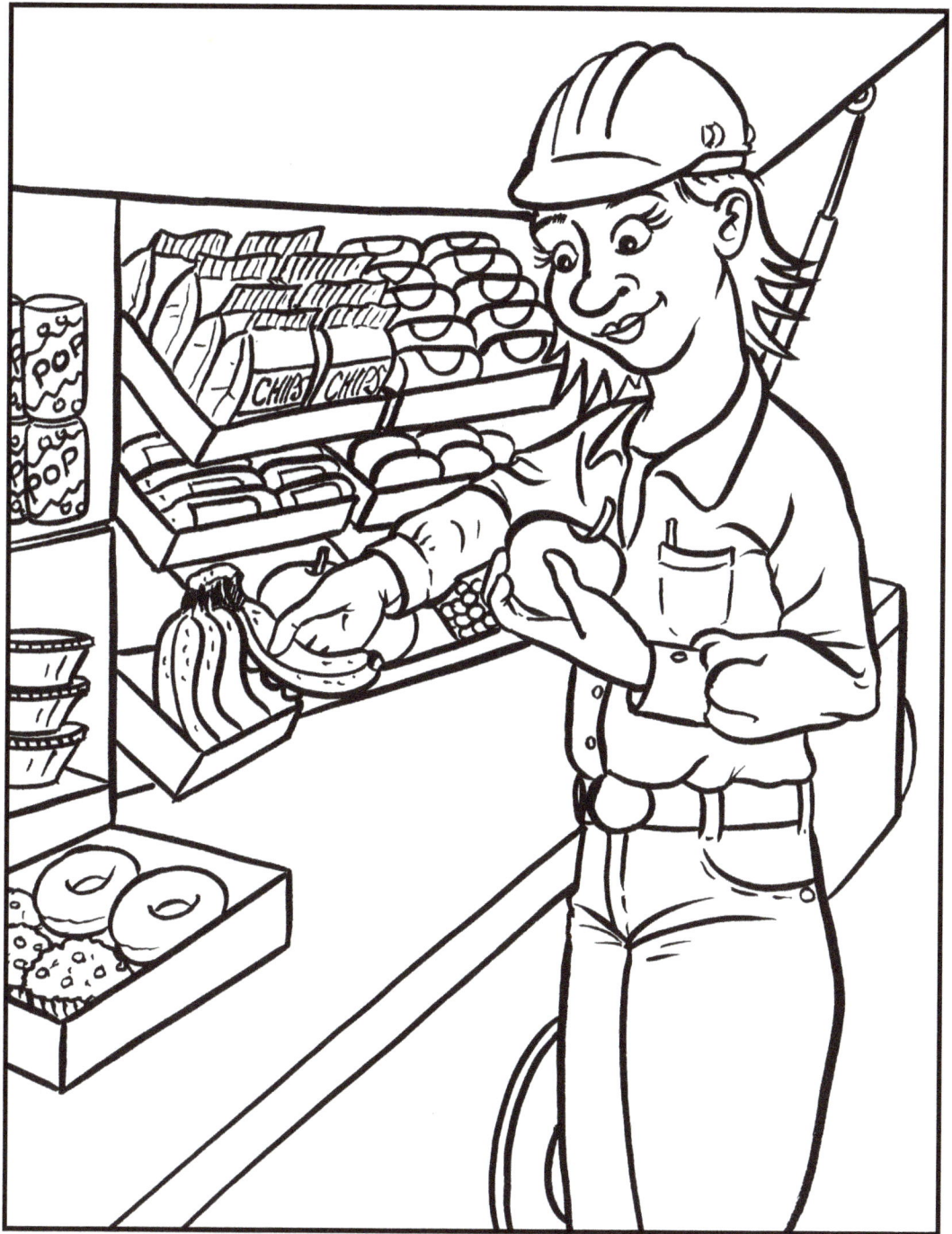

My mom knows how important a good night's sleep and healthy food and drink can affect how she thinks and acts.

Mi mamá sabe que una buena noche de sueño y alimentos y bebidas saludables pueden afectar su manera de pensar y actuar.

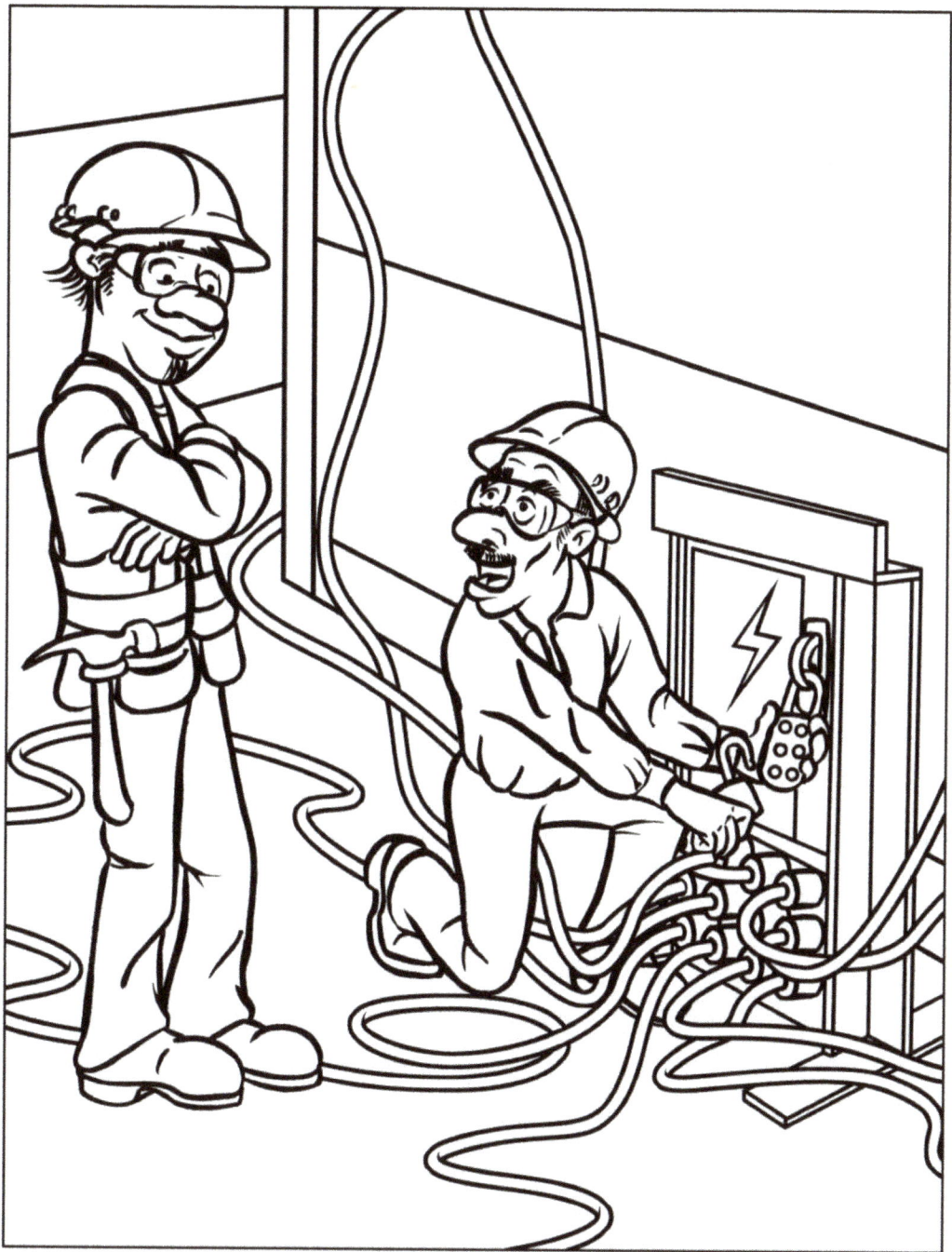

When dealing with electrical stuff, my brother always checks with
an electrician just to be sure not to be in any danger.

*Cuando se trata de las cosas eléctricas, mi hermano siempre consulta
con el electricista para estar seguro de no correr ningún peligro.*

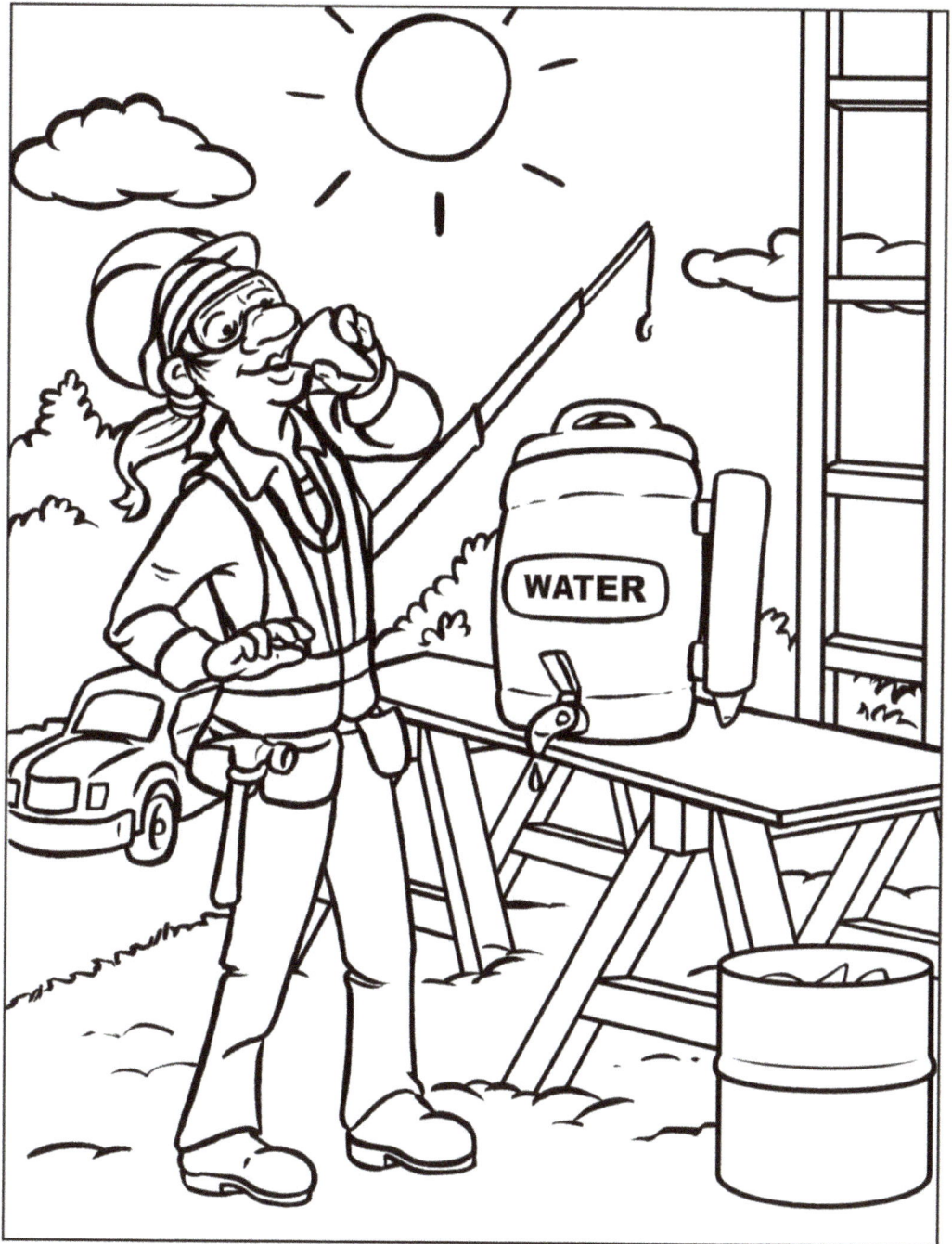

When it's hot outside, my sister always
drinks plenty of water.

Cuando hace calor, mi hermana siempre bebe mucha agua.

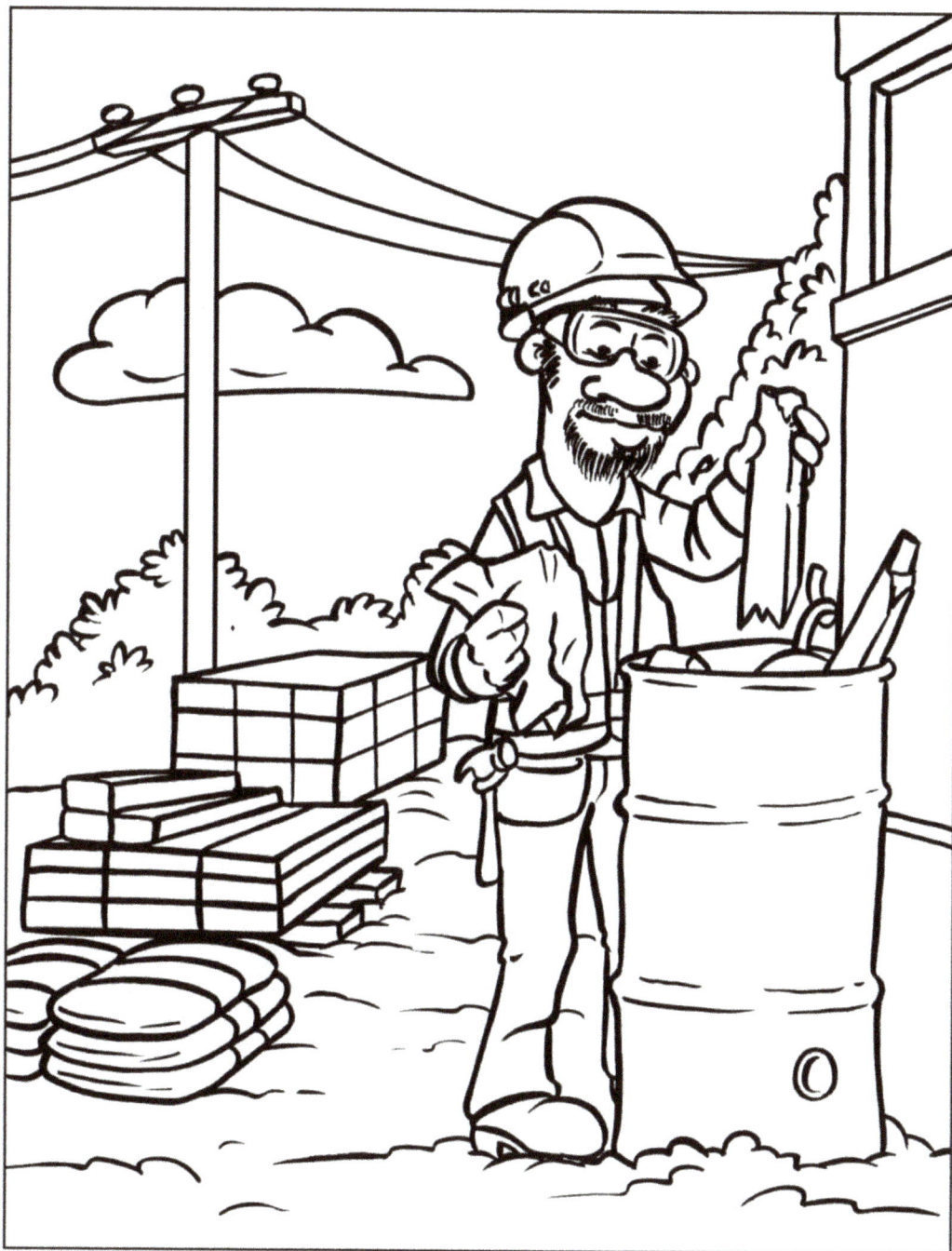

My uncle says that when the jobsite is clean,
it is much safer at work.

*Mi tío dice que en el trabajo hay más seguridad
cuando está limpia la obra.*

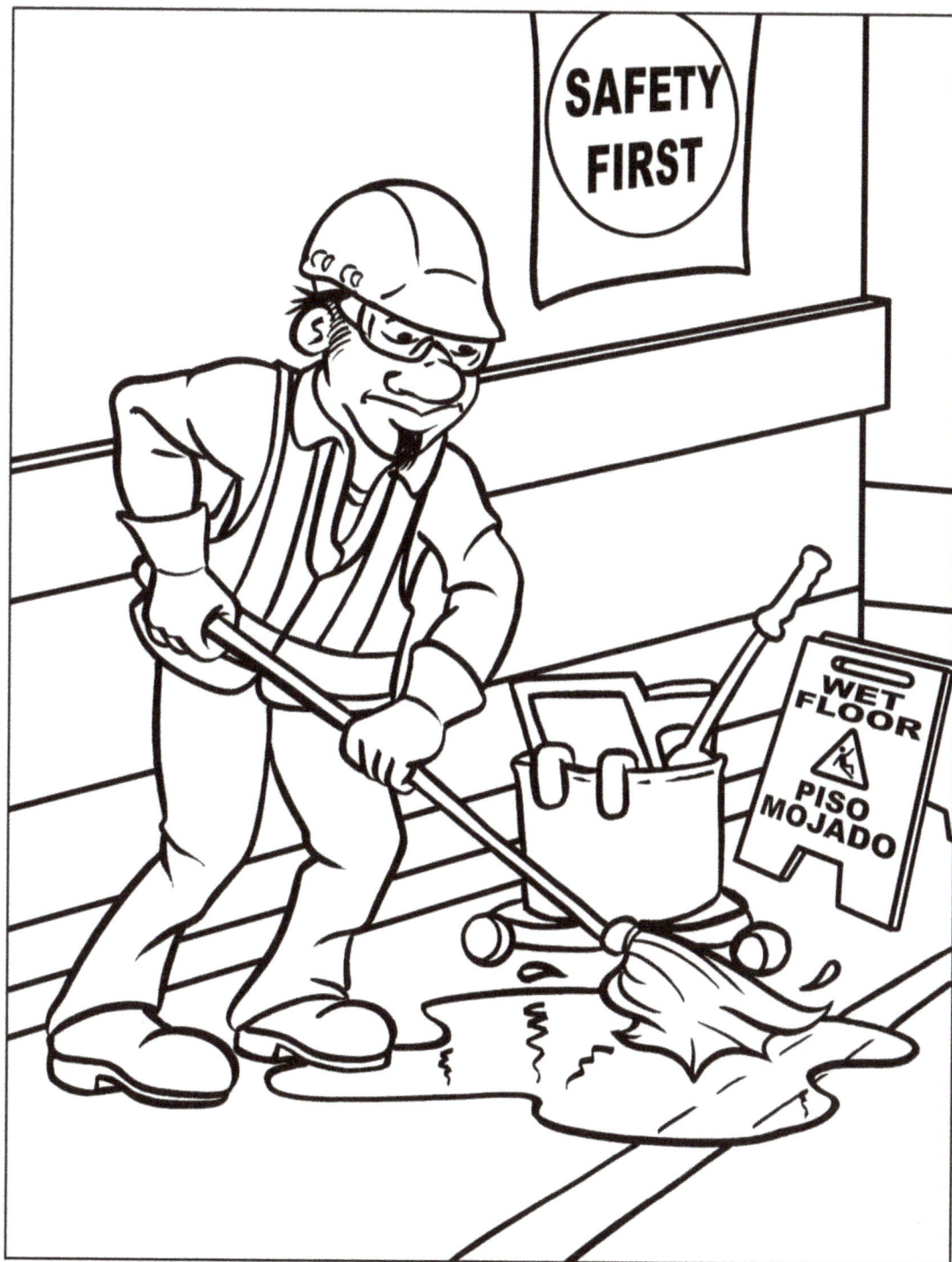

My brother cleans up any spills so that no one will slip.

*Mi hermano limpia cualquier derrame que hay
para que no se resbale nadie.*

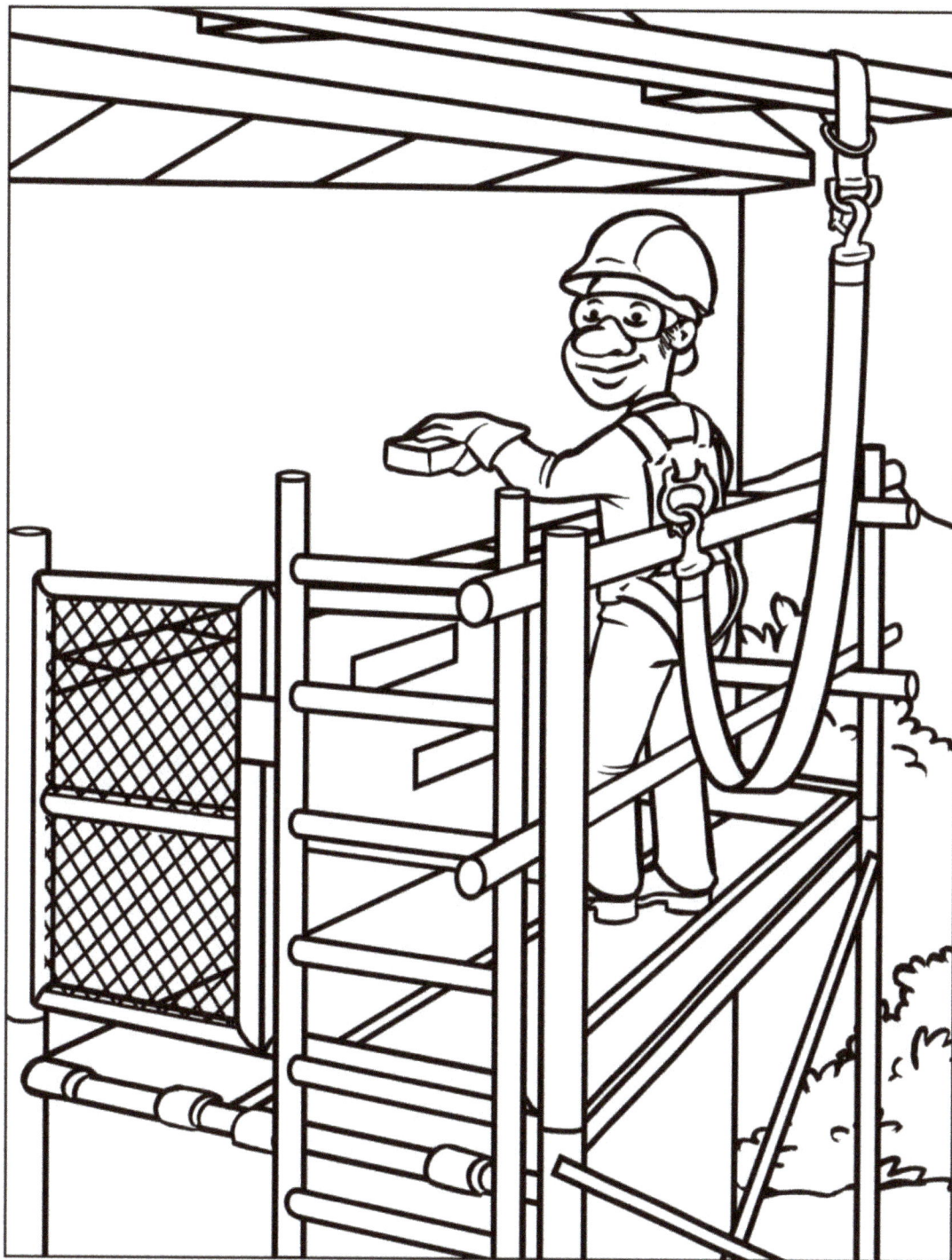

My dad always wears a full safety harness and ties himself
off when he's working over six feet off the ground.

*Mi papá siempre se pone el arnés completo y se amarra con las correas
de seguridad si trabaja a una altura de más de seis pies por encima del piso.*

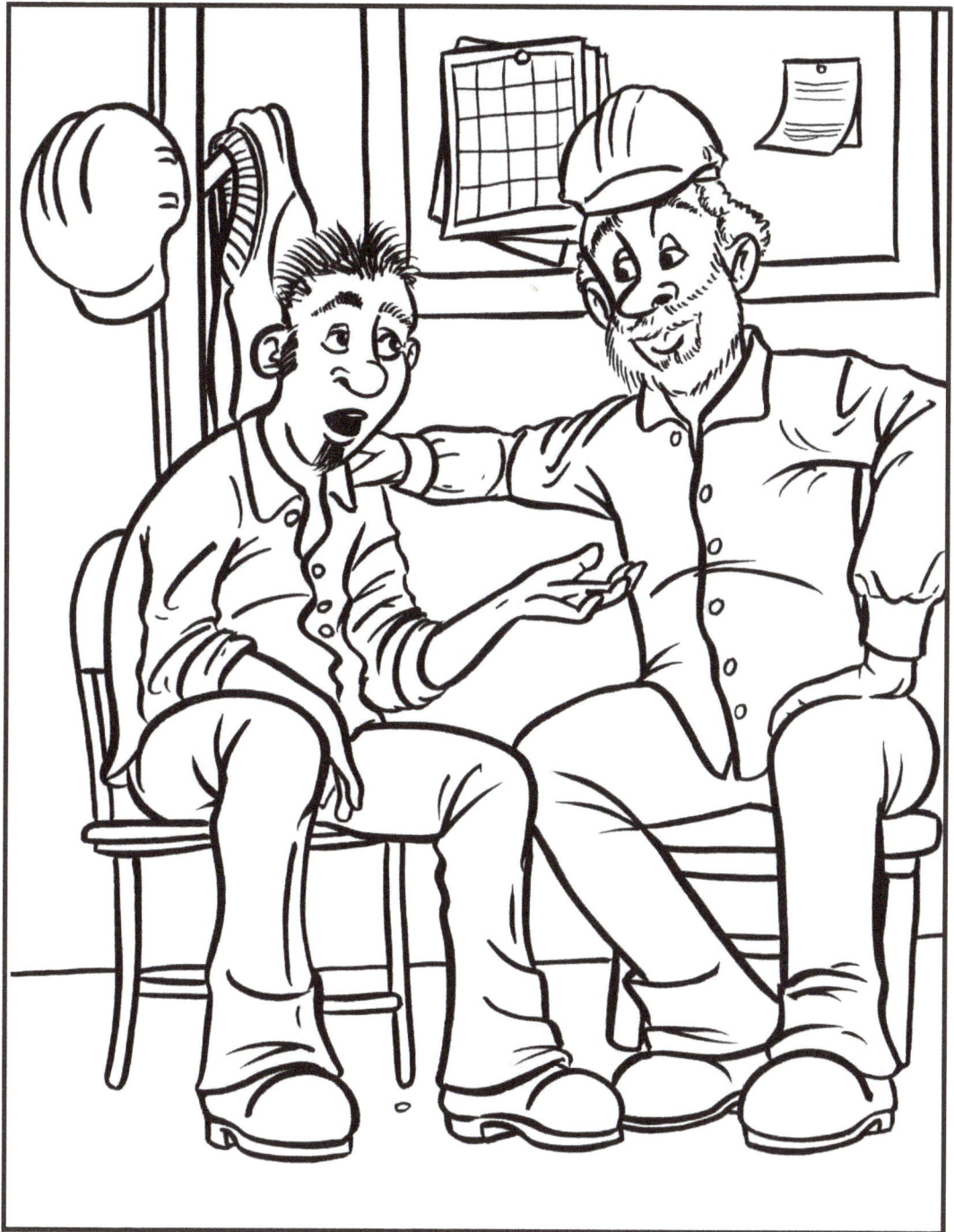

My brother knows that mental health is just as important as physical health and talks to his best friend on the project when he is feeling overwhelmed.

Mi hermano sabe que la salud mental es tan importante como la salud física y habla con su mejor amigo en el proyecto cuando se siente abrumado.

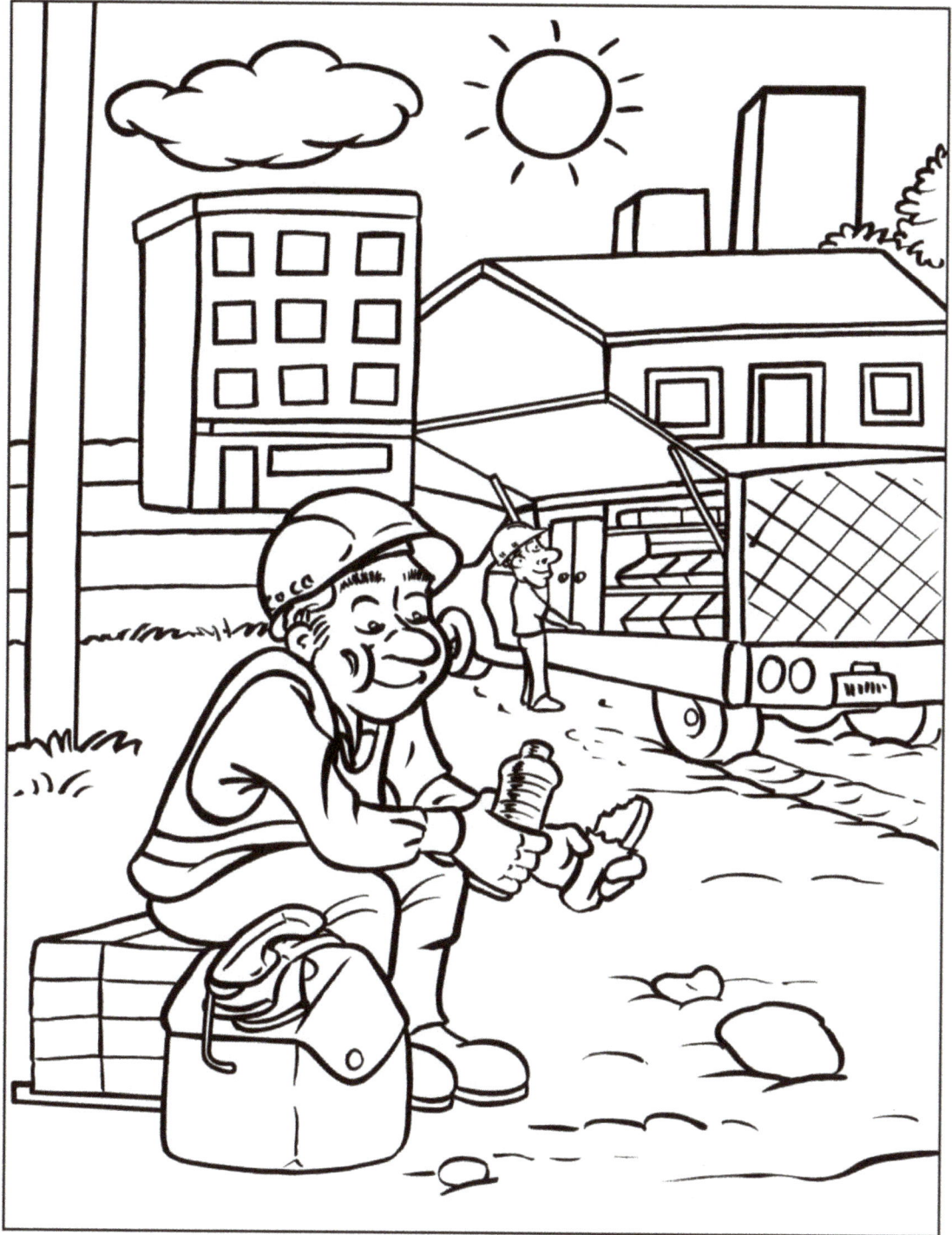

My dad knows when he is tired and takes a break.
People can have an accident when they work when they're tired.

*Mi papá lo sabe cuando se siente cansado, y se toma un descanso,
pues puede haber un accidente si la gente trabaja cuando está cansada.*

17

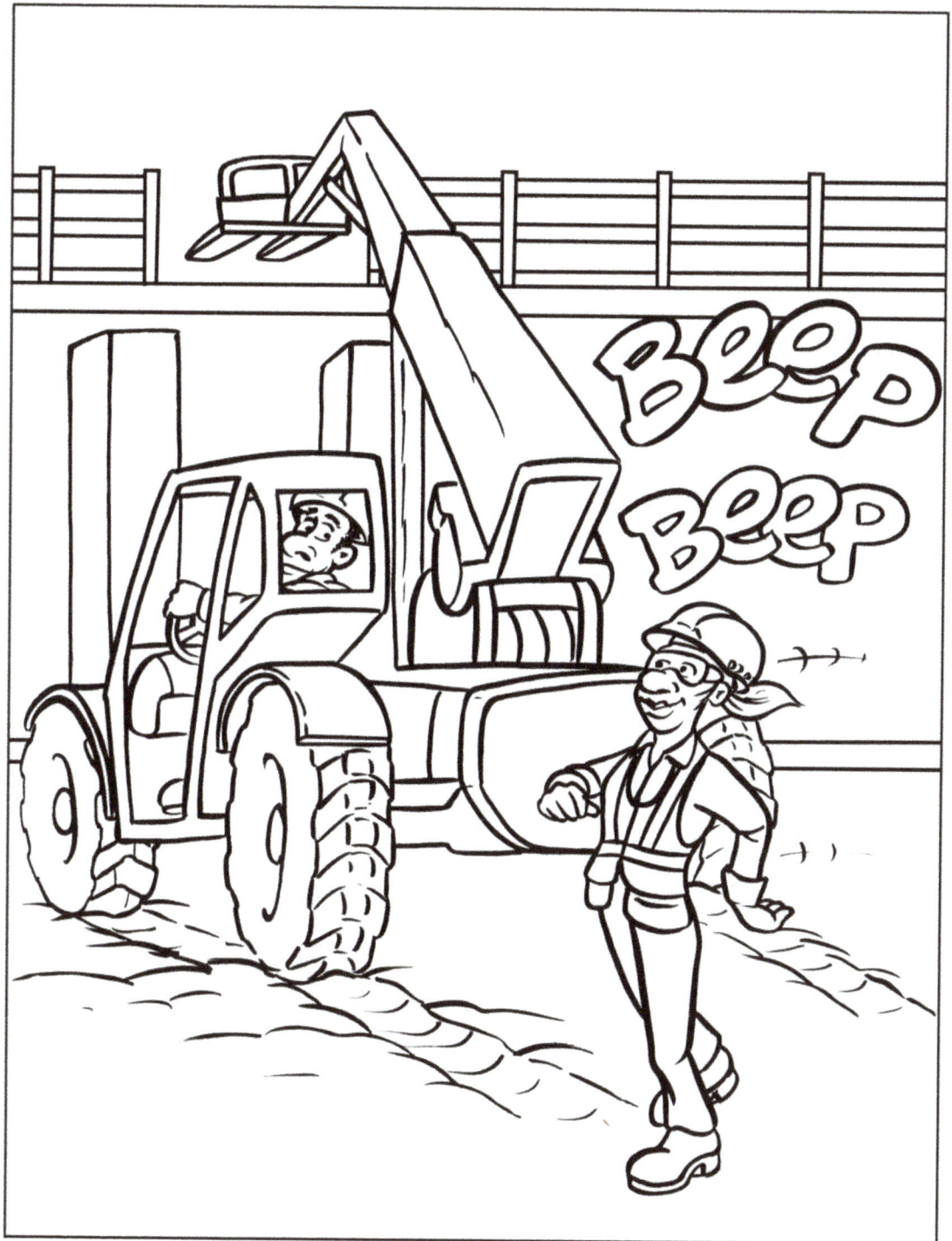

When my sister hears a backup alarm,
she gets out of the way.

*Si mi hermana escucha la bocina de marcha atrás,
se pone de un lado.*

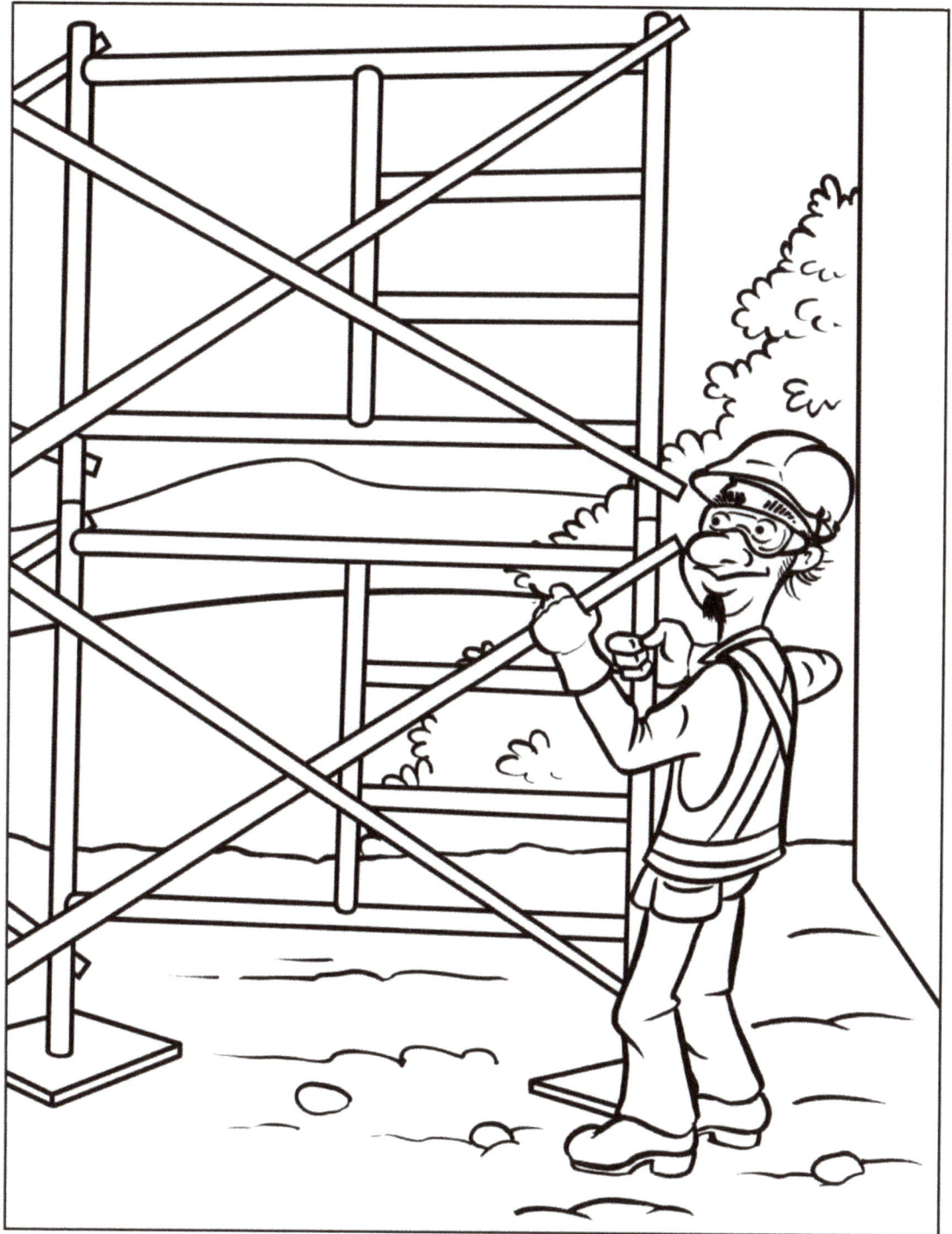

My brother makes sure that the ladders
and scaffolds are safe.

*Mi hermano se asegura que estén con la seguridad adecuada
las escaleras y los andamios.*

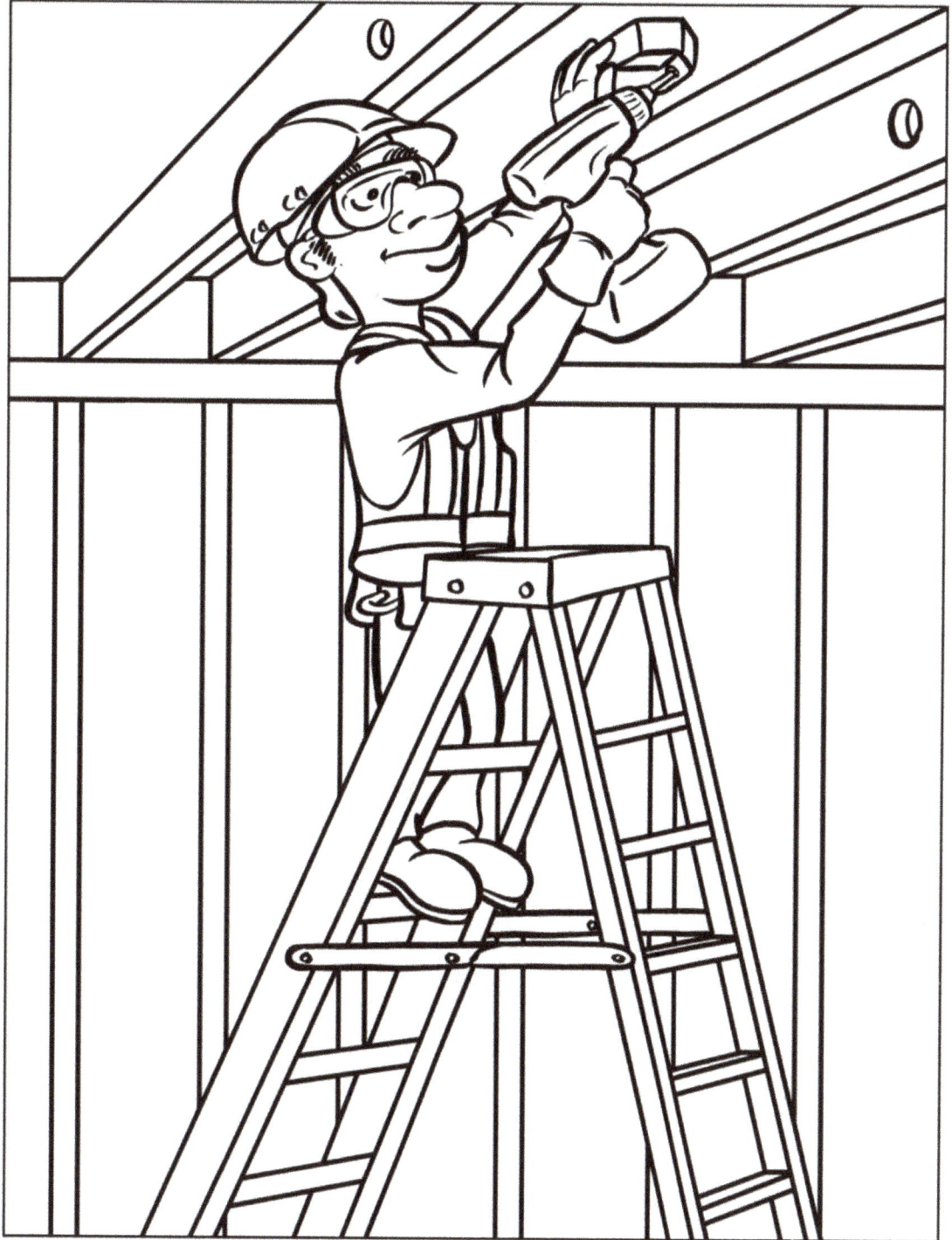

My dad never works on the top step of a ladder.
He stays safely on the lower steps.

*Mi papá nunca se sube en el último peldaño de la
escalera para trabajar, pues se queda en los peldaños
de más abajo para la seguridad.*

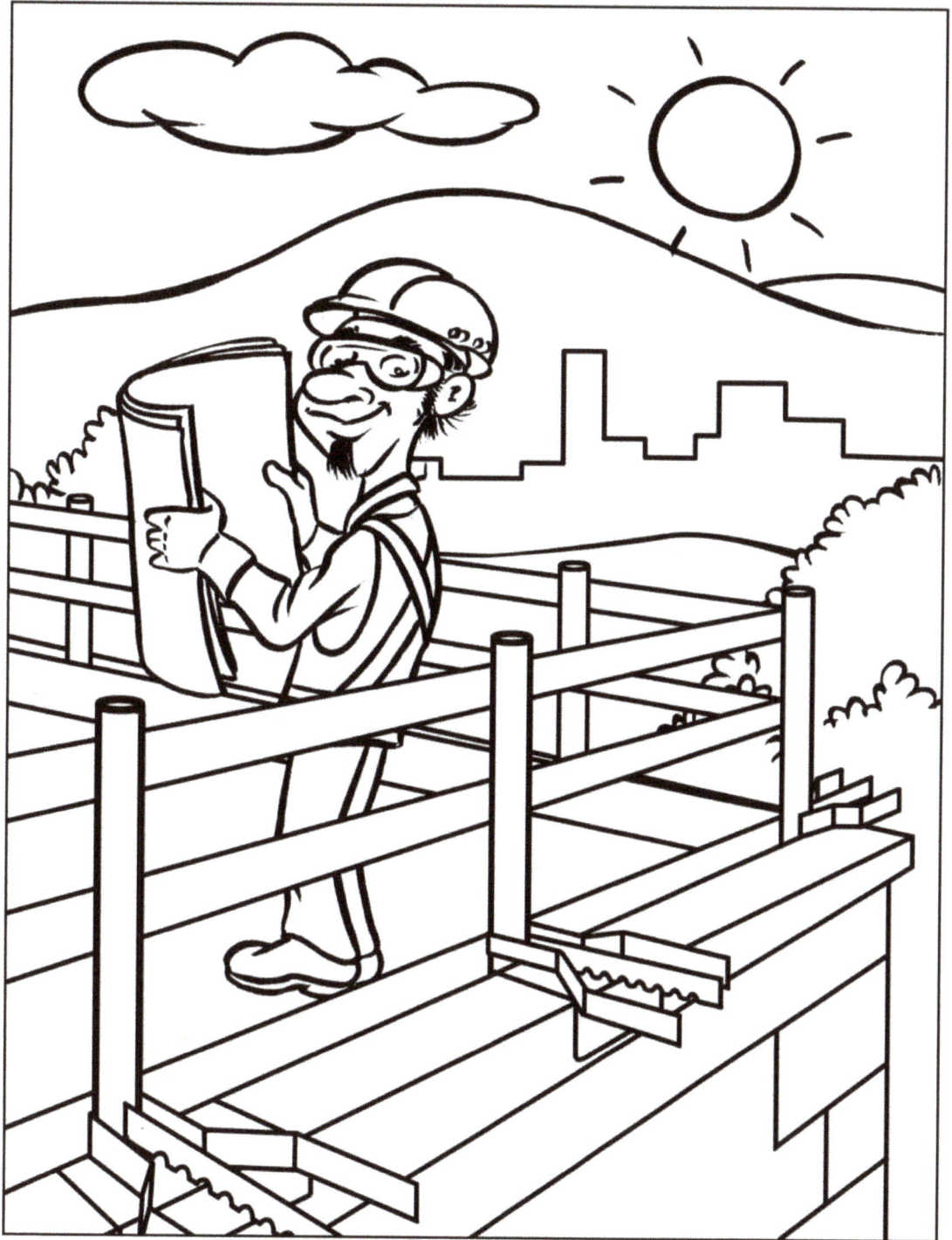

My brother never works in a high area without handrails.

*Mi hermano no trabaja nunca en una zona con altura,
a menos que haya alguna barandilla.*

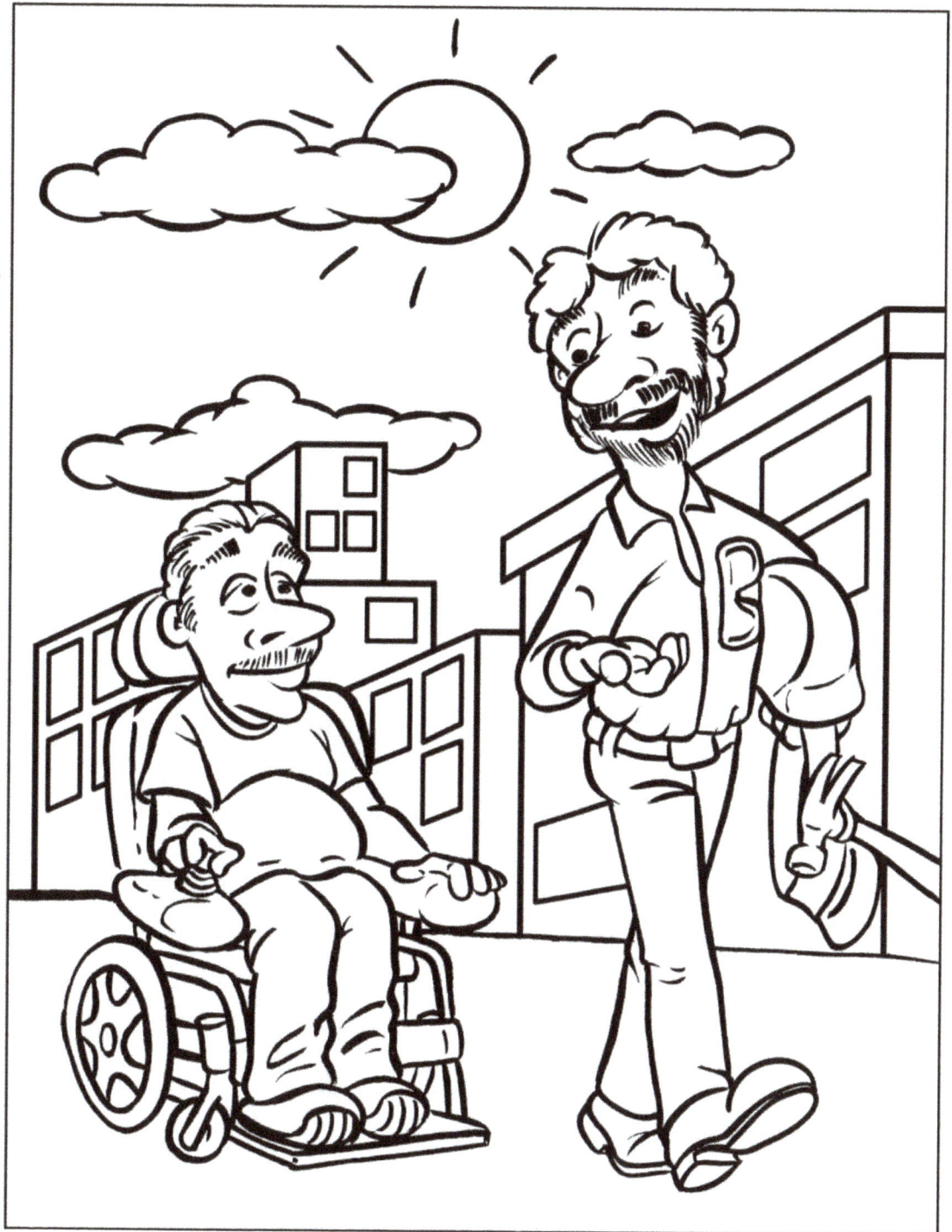

My uncle knows someone who didn't use his safety harness,
and he fell, and now he is in a wheelchair.

*Mi tío conoce a alguien que no usó el arnés de seguridad,
pues se cayó y ahora está en una silla de ruedas.*

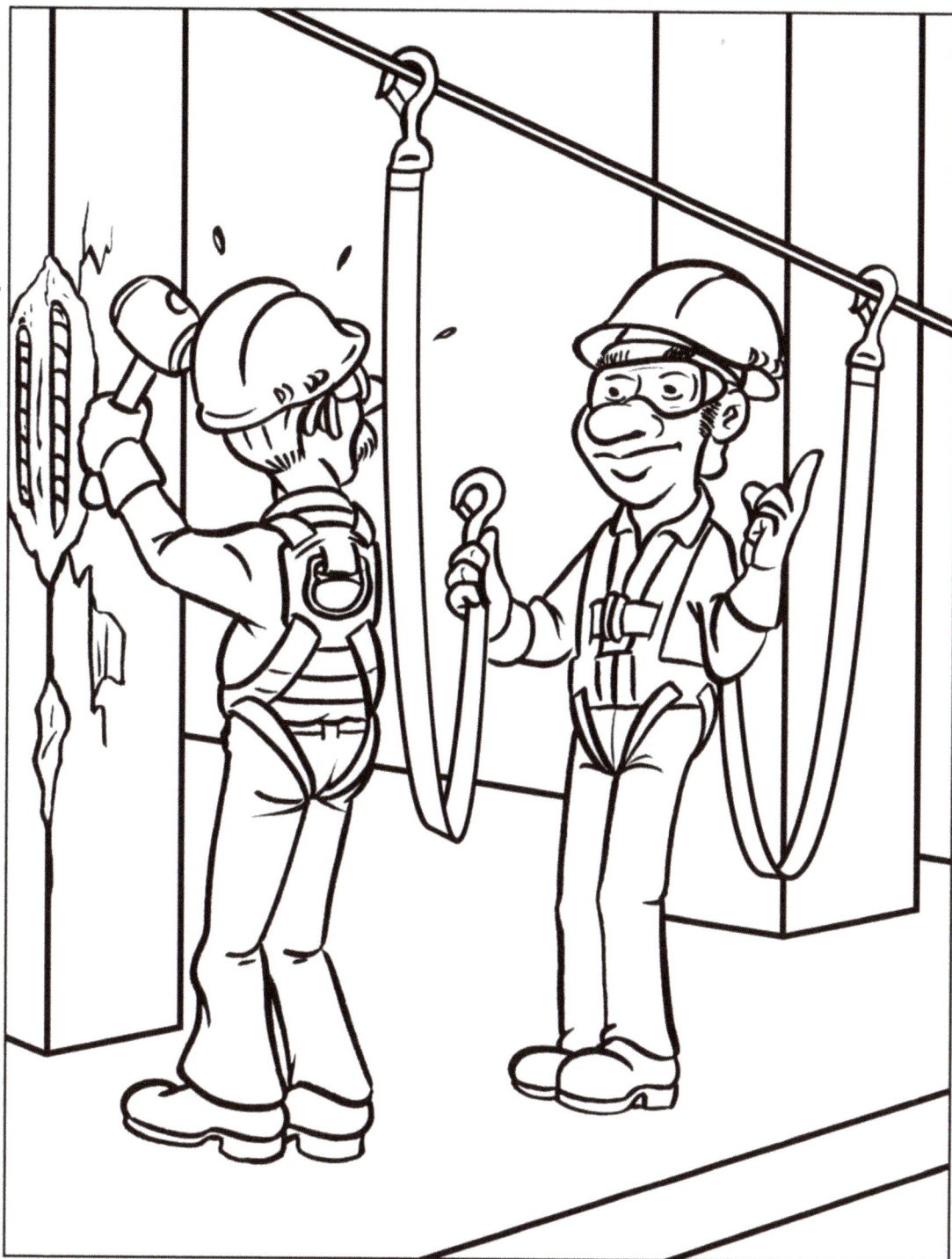

If my dad sees someone not working safely, he points it out.

*Mi papá se lo dice si ve a alguien que está trabajando
sin la seguridad indicada.*

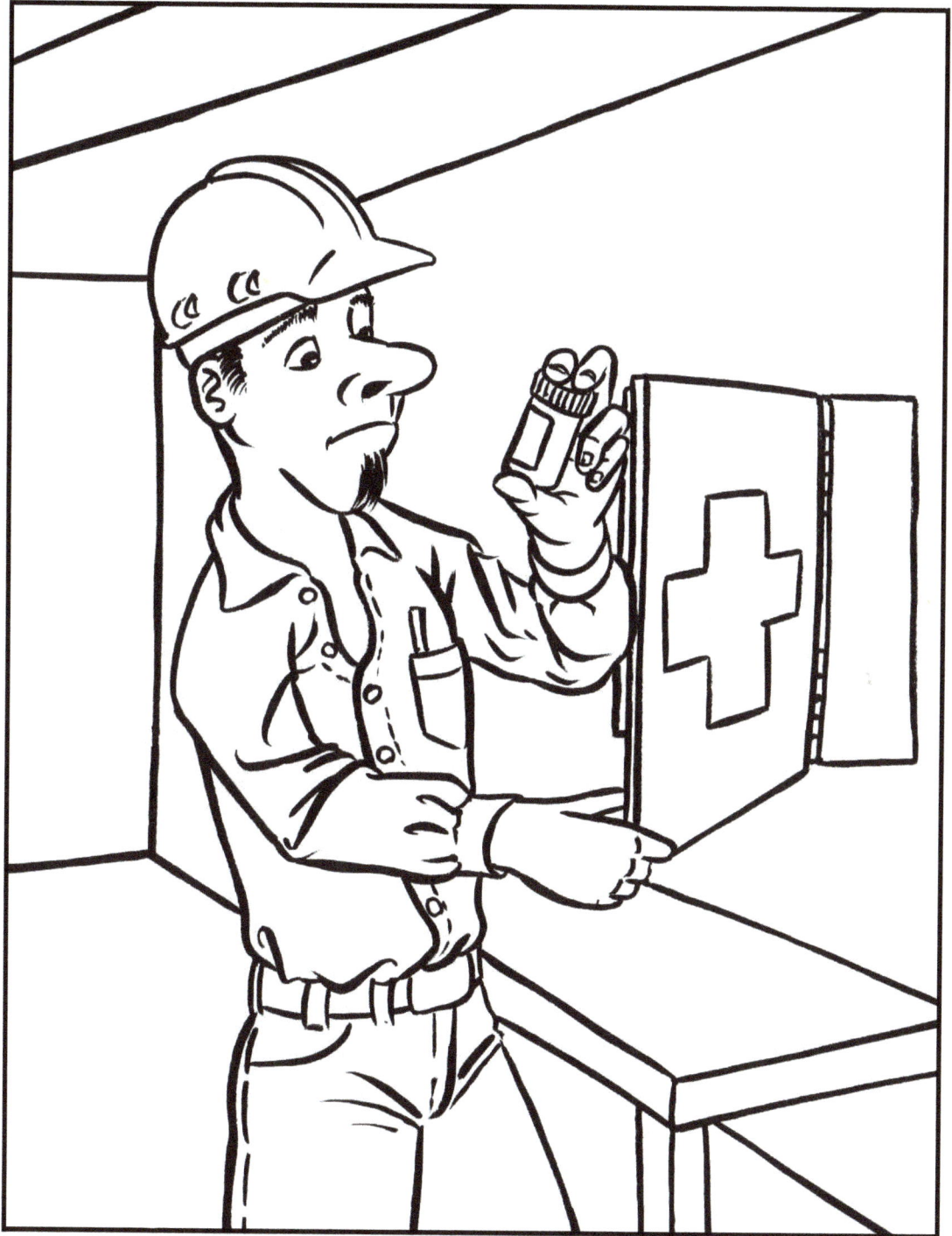

My brother is very aware of how drugs and medications,
even over the counter ones, can negatively affect how safely he works.

*Mi hermano es muy consciente de cómo las drogas y los medicamentos, incluso los de venta
libre, pueden afectar negativamente su funcionamiento.*

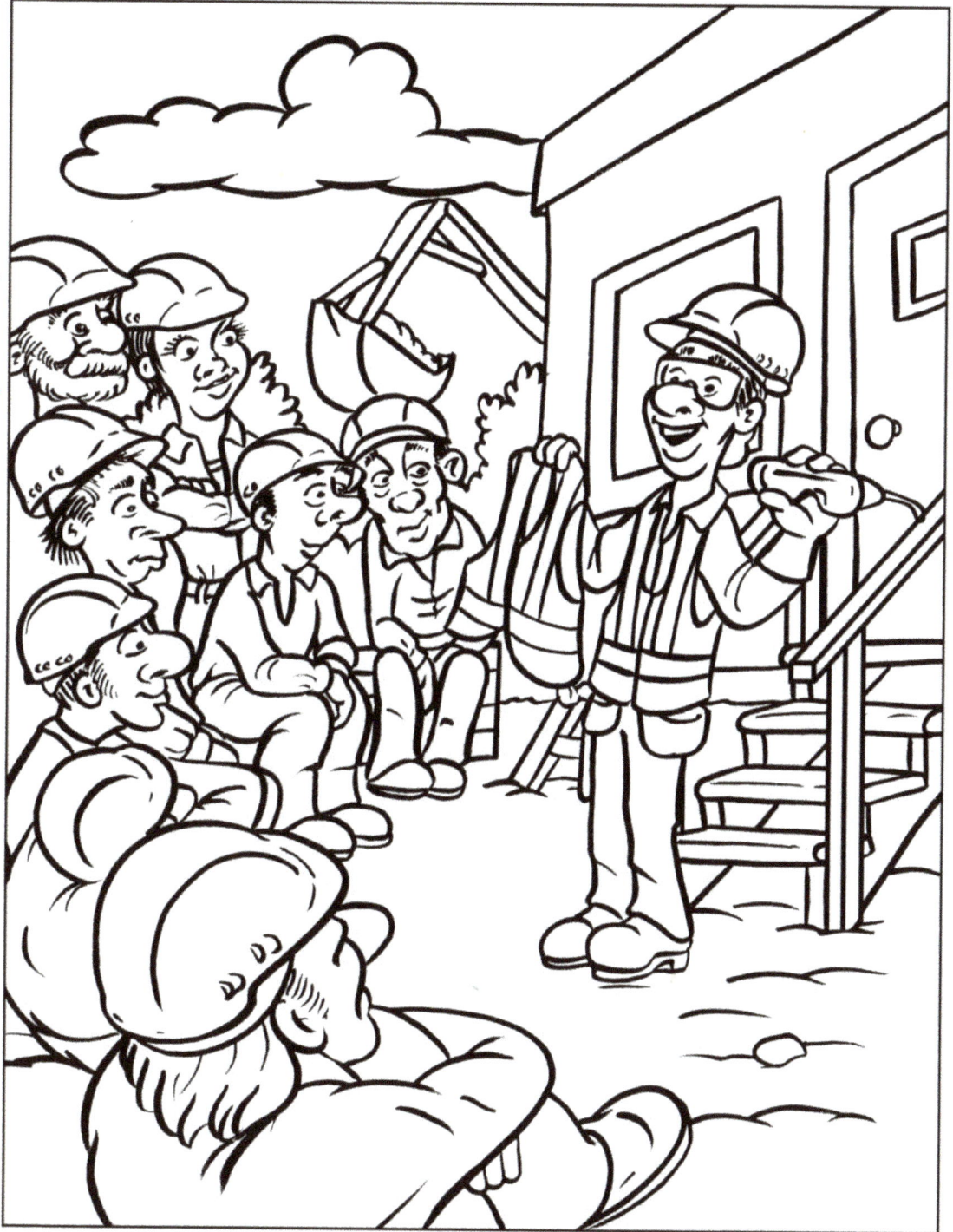

When we care about each other, we work more safely.
It takes all of us to work safely on a jobsite.

Cuando nos preocupamos el uno por el otro, trabajamos con más seguridad.
Necesitamos a todos nosotros para trabajar con seguridad en un sitio de trabajo.

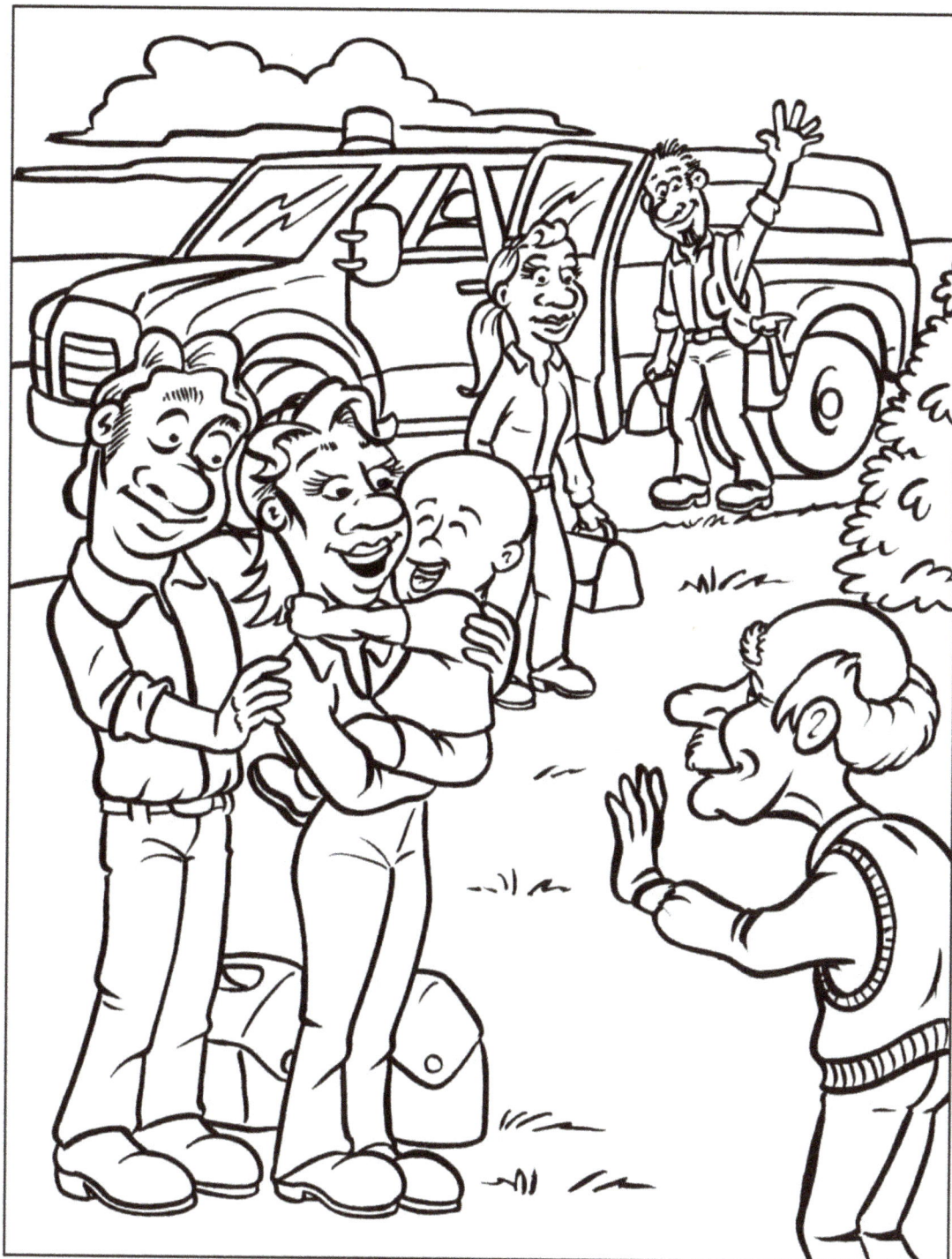

Working safely means that
my family comes home to me each night.

*El trabajar con la seguridad quiere decir que mi familia regresa
del trabajo todas las noches a estar conmigo.*

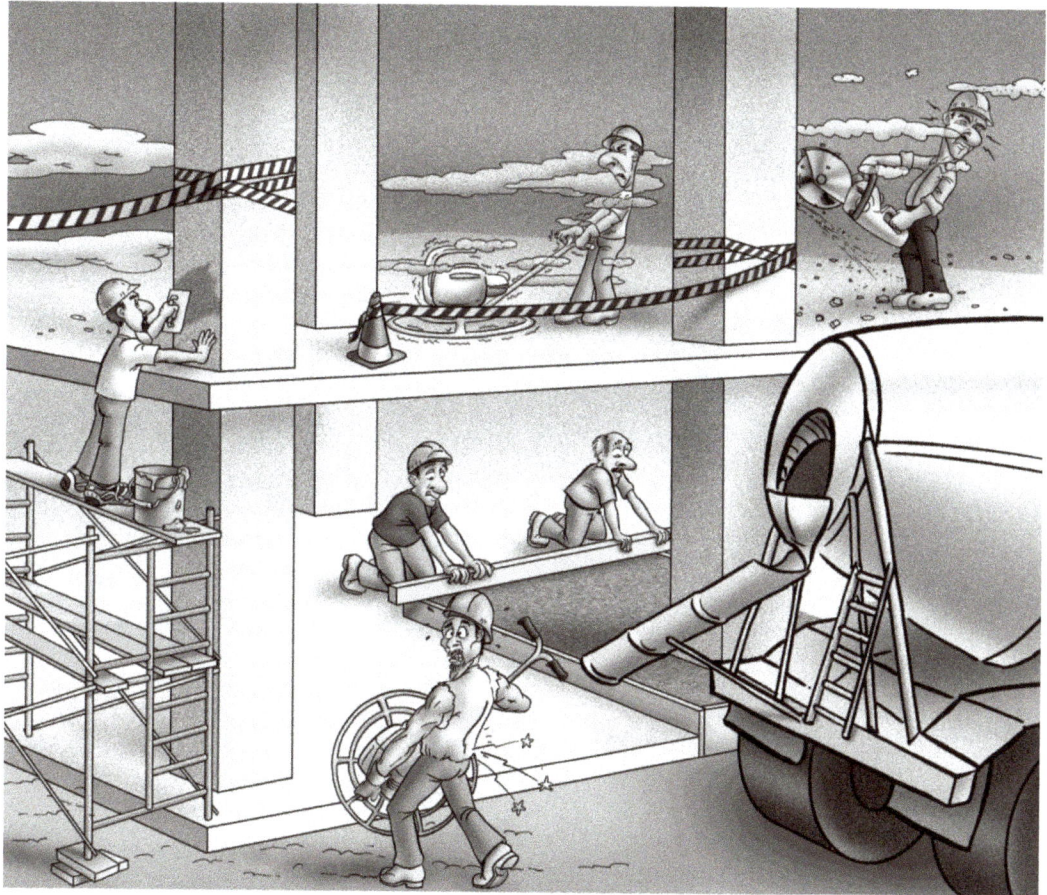

There are people in this picture not working safely.
Can you find the things that are wrong?

*Algunas de las personas en este dibujo trabajan sin la seguridad.
¿Puedes encontrar lo que está mal?*

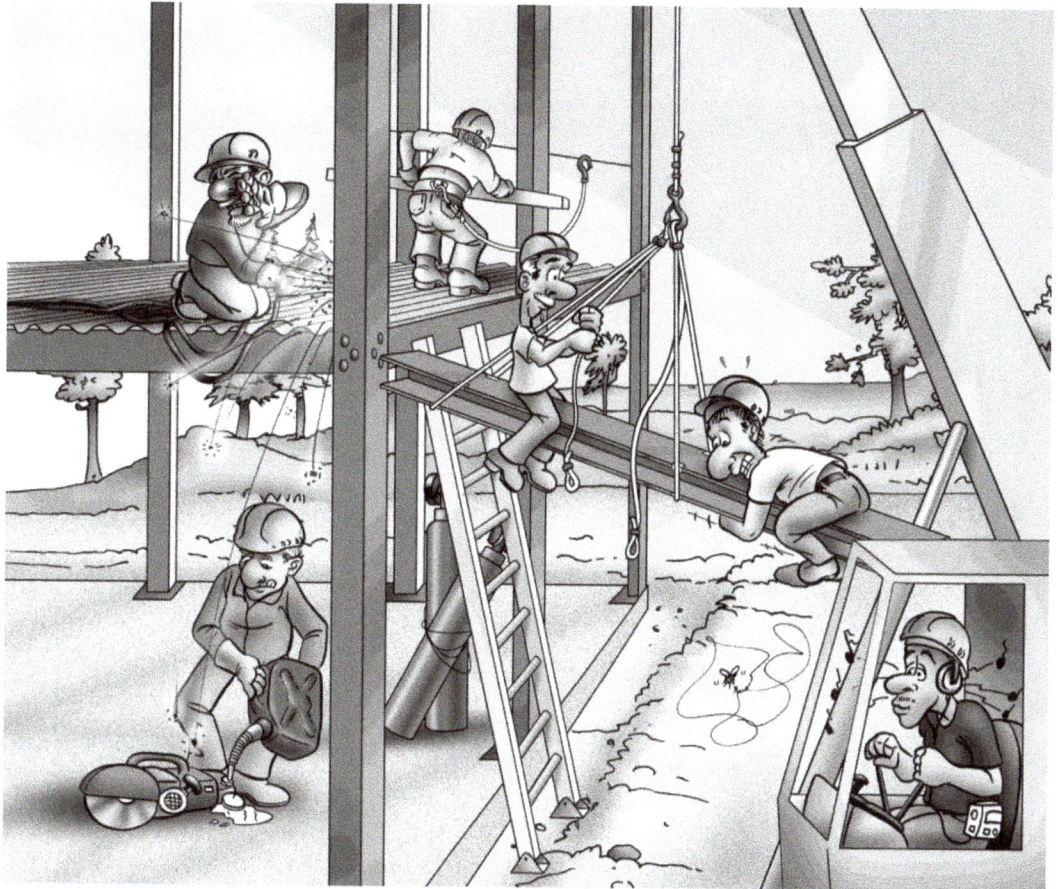

There are people in this picture not working safely.
Can you find the things that are wrong?

*Algunas de las personas en este dibujo trabajan sin la seguridad.
¿Puedes encontrar lo que está mal?*

Primal Safety Toolbox Safety Topics

The toolbox safety meetings should be fun and informative. You should not only discuss best safety practices, rules, and regulations, but address the emotional side of safety as well. We recommend walking safety meetings and mini-safety meetings. Walk around in large or small groups and point out safety issues like housekeeping, working from heights, scaffold and ladder safety, barriers and handrails, personal protective equipment, and any other safety topics that you find to be relevant. Ask them for their input. Ask them what they see. Ask them to point out what is wrong.

Stretch every morning. Have some theme from Rocky or James Brown I Feel Good playing.

Pair up. Have everyone introduce themselves and tell about their family (whatever that definition is for them).

Pair up. Get back to back. Remove a piece of safety equipment. Face each other and see if you can guess what is missing.

Get in small groups and discuss the potential dangers for the day and how to overcome them.

Walk around in small groups and have everyone point out potentially unsafe areas and situations.

Celebrate everyone's birthday for each month and give each person a small gift. At lunch, have a big sheet cake for everyone.

Pair up. Tell each other why it's important that you go home safely that day.

Tell a story about a near miss or a save and what it meant to that person.

Hand out Primal Safety Coloring books and crayons. Have their kids color the pages, laminate the pages and put them up around the project.

Discuss the importance of glucose in your brain and decision making.

Tell everyone to take five deep breaths and relax. A non-stressed brain makes better decisions.

Pair up. Tell each other a lifelong dream that you have.

Pair up. Tell each other a family story.

Pair up. Ask each other, "Why is it important that you work safely?"

Pair up. Tell each other what would happen if they went to work today without any personal protective equipment on.

Discuss how stress shuts down your thinking brain and keeps you from making good decisions.

Hand out some healthy snacks for the day like some nuts or healthy protein bars.

Show the group an unsafe situation or scenario and see if they can come up with an intervention and solution. Make it a contest.

Actually show how a harness can protect against a fall.

Tell everyone how dehydration affects them: Increased thirst, dry mouth, swollen tongue, weakness, dizziness, palpitations, confusion, sluggishness, fainting, no sweat, decreased urine.

Celebrate a safety milestone with a short party with food.

Read an obituary from someone who died on a construction project and what family was left behind.

Have everyone take the Ghyst EI Test and discuss how their profile can affect safety.

Tell them that if they are working unsafely, you will send them home and they can't return until they have a note from their spouse or family member.

Discuss how their judgment can be impaired from lack of sleep.

Discuss how their judgment can be impaired from drugs (OTC, prescription, recreational).

Discuss how good nutrition will not only positively affect performance, but they will also live a longer, healthier life.

Discuss why they are so tired at the end of the day: poor nutrition, poor sleep, not enough breaks, dehydration, holding muscles in tension, distracted thoughts, energy vampires (people who suck the life out of you). Also discuss how you can reduce these.

Discuss safety and alpha males and how this hypermasculine environment is not good for safety. A caring environment yields much better safety and productivity numbers.

Have everyone tell how they celebrate Holidays.

Have everyone tell how they celebrate birthdays.

Have everyone tell how they celebrate becoming an adult.

Tap into a larger purpose for your project and create a family work environment where everyone values and cares for each other.

Have everyone tell about how their kids reacted to The Primal Safety Coloring Book.

Have everyone tell each other that they want them to go home safely today.

Pair off. Tell each other how you overcame a struggle during childhood.

Have everyone jump up and down 10 times. Get the energy up for a safe day.

Have everyone discuss how their mental state (stressed, angry, etc) affects safety.

Have everyone discuss the importance of taking breaks.

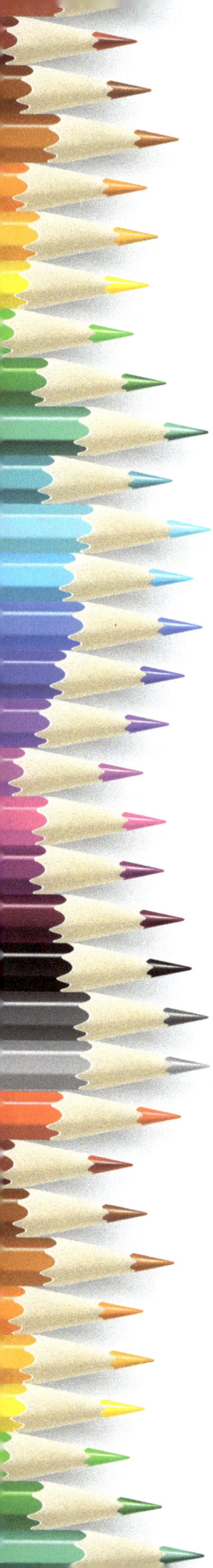

Have everyone discuss the importance of not working while tired or hungry.

Discuss how mobile phones can be distracting and unsafe while working.

Use mobile phones during the meeting to call or text a loved one and let them know that you will work safely that day.

Discuss how safety can increase productivity.

Discuss how organization and cleanup can affect attitudes and safety.

Have everyone get into small groups and tell a joke or good story.

Show what multi-tasking is a myth. It's really multi-switching and it is not good for high levels of safety. Tell them to count to 24by 2s. Then spell multitasking. Time each one. Then tell them to alternate them: 2, m, 4, u, 6, l, etc. Time that. It usually takes two to three times longer.

Have everyone shut their eyes and do a visualization of a safe day and what it looks like.

Pair off. Have everyone tell a story about the kids in their life.

Pair off. Have everyone tell a story about how they met their spouse or partner. If they don't have a partner, tell them to tell a story about how they met their best friend.

Have a discussion on what family means and what it means to look out for each other.

Pair off. Have everyone discuss how they would teach their kids about how to use their personal protective equipment.

Have a discussion about a future vision such as their life five years from now or when they retire and what they hope to accomplish.

PRIMAL SAFETY:
A GUT LEVEL APPROACH

We have developed a safety program called Primal Safety®. This unique program states that everyone has the basic human right to go home alive and free from injuries at the end of the day. But with that right comes the responsibility to watch out for each other, to care for each other enough to point out unsafe situations, and to take the necessary corrective actions.

Employees and project teams focus on emotional competencies such as emotional self-awareness, empathy, and interpersonal relationship skills. Key team members take the EQ-i® 2.0 and develop the areas that are required for a successful program. Employees and project teams form closer relationships with each other with a deliberate approach to relationship building. Employees and project teams learn about each other's lives outside of work. This is done both formally and informally through activities for the workers and their families. Family members and loved ones become part of the safety process. Employees and project teams develop a greater awareness of safety – not because of rules but because the workers will care enough about each other to keep each other safe.

Primal Safety® program specifics:

The purpose of this program is to enhance the safety program that you already have in place.

The project team and any other appropriate parties take the Emotional Quotient Inventory (EQ-i® 2.0). We also have a free EI test available. This measures their emotional self-awareness, empathy, social responsibility, and interpersonal relationships. Without this foundation, typical construction EI profiles will likely limit the effectiveness of this program. One of the highest competencies measured by the EQ-i® 2.0 for construction folks is independence. Most of the folks in the industry defy death daily, working in a dangerous environment. It's like NASCAR drivers or bullfighters. There is an element of danger in what they do, and they are not fearful of death. But with high levels of independence, most have the fear of being dependent on others. If you tell them to work safely or die, you may get a smile or shrug of a shoulder. But if you say to them, "If you don't work safely, your wife may be feeding you and wiping your bottom", they sit up and take notice.

The basic premise of the **Primal Safety®** program is that everyone in your company has a moral imperative to implement an effective safety program for all workers, including subcontractors, affording every worker the basic human right to go home each day uninjured to their family and loved ones. This means ZERO TOLERANCE! No accident or unsafe situation, no matter how small or insignificant, is acceptable. This approach is similar to how Bill Bratton, the former

New York police commissioner, cleaned up the city. It was called the "broken window" theory. When there was a broken window, it was replaced. When graffiti showed up, it was removed the same day. There was zero tolerance of the smallest of infractions, because if minor infractions were not addressed, it led to larger infractions and more serious crimes.

All employees are encouraged to report any accident, potential accident, or unsafe situation, no matter how small. Every report is acted upon. Blame is not assessed, violators are not punished, and reporters are thanked and encouraged. The process is as follows:

    a. Analyze why the hazardous situation exists.

    b. Correct the situation.

    c. Educate the violators as to the proper means and methods in the spirit of learning and improving.

    d. Communicate these reports to everyone in order to avoid this situation in the future.

As part of the safety orientation, all employees share their personal stories about how they have been affected by accidents.

All safety activities are tracked and recorded including accidents, avoided accidents, unsafe situations and behaviors, corrective actions, and communications. Everyone has access to this information, which is reinforced at all meetings.

There are numerous activities to reinforce these safety concepts. Some ideas:

    a. At meetings, where possible, everyone should say their name and what they think about any safety issues for that day. They should be asked probing questions as well. According to the book, The Checklist Manifesto, the simple act of saying your name and giving your input makes it much more likely that you will speak up when something isn't right. When people don't verbalize their name and give their input, they are far less likely to say anything, even if they perceive that something is wrong. If this is not possible for large meetings, break your safety meetings down to smaller groups. And don't forget to have interpreters if necessary.

    b. The toolbox safety meetings should be fun and informative. You should not only discuss best safety practices, rules, and regulations, but address the emotional side of safety as well. We recommend walking safety meetings and mini-safety meetings. Walk around in large or small groups and point out safety issues like housekeeping, working from heights, scaffold and ladder safety, barriers and handrails, personal protective equipment, and any other safety topics that you find to be relevant. Ask them for their input. Ask them what they see. Ask them to point out what is wrong. The Primal Safety Toolbox Safety Topics are in Appendix A.

    c. Each morning, the entire project team does five to ten minutes of calisthenics and warm-up exercises. This reinforces the team approach to safety and prevents accidents by getting the blood flowing, warming up

joints, and waking the team up mentally. We provide specific instructions to project team leaders on how to conduct this morning session. You may also use this session to highlight a safety issue for the day. According to a Swedish study on a construction project, morning warm-up exercises increased or maintained joint and muscle flexibility and muscle endurance for workers exposed to manual material handling and strenuous working positions. Over time, this will decrease the number of injuries and increase productivity.

d. Safety milestones are celebrated with jobsite lunches and team activities. These celebrations are also an opportunity to enhance the spirit of the team and create closer relationships among the workers.

e. There are social activities outside of work to encourage the workers to create closer relationships with each other. These may include sports activities, team sports, and other social activities.

f. Celebrations of birthdays, anniversaries, births, and other life milestones are encouraged. These celebrations reinforce the human side and put a face on safety.

g. A focus on quitting smoking and other tobacco use, good nutrition, weight loss, and exercise is a great way to let them know that you care about them as human beings. When they start implementing these concepts, their cognitive abilities will be increased. They will think more clearly, solve problems more readily, and work more safely.

h. Any way to remind them is beneficial. Everyone could wear reminder bands or stickers. Or everyone could wear pedometers if you started a walking or biggest loser contest on site.

There are family/social activities that reinforce safety. Some ideas:

a. All of the children of the workers make safety posters encouraging their parents to come home safely to them each day. The posters are laminated and placed throughout the project.

b. Put the photos of family members on hardhats along with their names. This will be a constant reminder of their loved ones and also create better relationships because everyone will be able to see your family and get to know them.

c. There are family days so that family members can visit the workplace and see demonstrations of the safety equipment that keeps their loved ones safe.

d. There are family social days such as picnics and parties. Every employee has someone who cares about his or her safety. Employees are not numbers. They are sons, daughters, fathers, mothers, brothers, and sisters. Find out which relationships matter the most for each employee.

e. Workers are encouraged to take their safety equipment home and show their families how this equipment protects them from getting hurt on the job.

f. Families are involved in the safety process. If there is a habitual violator, the family can be called in to help motivate that worker. This type of intervention has the potential to save lives.

g. Many projects now have webcams for security and also to check in on the project from remote locations. What if you started a campaign where you gave the families the web address so that they could look in on their loved ones while they were working? You could post signs that say, "Work safely. Your family is watching you."

THE FUTURE OF SAFETY: Where do you go after you reach zero accidents?

For a moment, look to the future and see a vision where the AEC industry is not only a safe industry, but actually becomes restorative. Imagine people working in this industry for years and retiring not only free from disabilities, but healthy and full of vigor. That is the next step in this process. Some say it is impossible to achieve. Some use the excuse that "this is a dangerous industry". Although there is no doubt that the work is tough and dangerous, we firmly believe that we can reach that level of health and safety through this emotionally intelligent approach and a true focus on people and their health and well-being. This will also address our poor industry image and workforce development issues. When we create this type of caring environment, people will flock to the industry.

www.ingramcontent.com/pod-product-compliance
Lightning Source LLC
Chambersburg PA
CBHW081722270326

41933CB00017B/3265